MOSBY'S
Medical Terminology
Memory
NoteCards

Visual, Mnemonic, and Memory
Aids for Healthcare Professionals

JoAnn Zerwekh, EdD, RN, FNP, APRN, BC

Executive Director
Nursing Education Consultants
Ingram, Texas

Nursing Faculty – Online Campus
University of Phoenix
Phoenix, Arizona

Tom Gaglione, RN, MSN
Nurse Consultant
Kerrville, Texas

C.J. Miller, BSN, RN
Illustrator
Nursing Education Consultants
Washington, Iowa

Reviewed by
Betsy J. Shiland, MS, RHIA, CPHQ, CTR
Ashley Zerwekh, RN, MS

MOSBY
ELSEVIER

MOSBY
ELSEVIER

11830 Westline Industrial Drive
St. Louis, Missouri 63146

MOSBY'S MEDICAL TERMINOLOGY
MEMORY NOTECARDS: VISUAL,
MNEMONIC, AND MEMORY AIDS
FOR HEALTHCARE PROFESSIONALS

ISBN-13: 978-0-323-04567-4

Library of Congress Control Number: 2007929359

Executive Publisher: Andrew Allen
Publisher: Jeanne Wilke
Senior Developmental Editor: Linda Woodard
Publishing Services Manager: Pat Joiner-Myers
Senior Project Manager: Karen M. Rehwinkel
Designer: Kim Denando
Cover Art: CJ Miller

Printed in China

Last digit is the print number: 9 8 7 6 5 4 3 2 1

Contents

INTRODUCTION TO BASIC TERMINOLOGY

ANATOMICAL, POSITIONAL, AND DIRECTIONAL TERMS

BODY CAVITIES

CELLS: HUMAN BUILDING BLOCKS

CONGENITAL DISORDERS

DISCIPLINES

BODY SYSTEMS AND MAIN STRUCTURES

Contents

TYPES OF DISEASES

DIAGNOSTIC PROCEDURES

PHARMACOLOGY

DON'T CONFUSE THESE!

Use your *Memory Notecards* with any of these trusted textbooks for a complete understanding of medical terminology!

The Language of Medicine, 8th Edition
Davi-Ellen Chabner, BA, MAT
ISBN: 978-1-4160-3492-6

Exploring Medical Language, 6th Edition
Myrna LaFleur Brooks, BEd, RN, CHUC
ISBN: 978-0-323-02805-9

Quick & Easy Medical Terminology, 5th Edition
Peggy C. Leonard, BA, MT, MEd
ISBN: 978-1-4160-2494-1

Mastering Healthcare Terminology, 2nd Edition
Betsy J. Shiland, MS, RHIA, CPHQ, CTR
ISBN: 978-0-323-03572-9

Get your copies today!

- Order online at www.elsevierhealth.com
- Visit your local bookstore
- Call Customer Service toll-free at 1-800-545-2522

HP-07112

FINALLY, MEDICAL TERMINOLOGY MADE CLEAR! USE YOUR NEW MEDICAL TERMINOLOGY NOTECARDS AS A:

- Companion study guide for medical terminology texts
- Quick review for examinations
- Reference to use with other health care texts

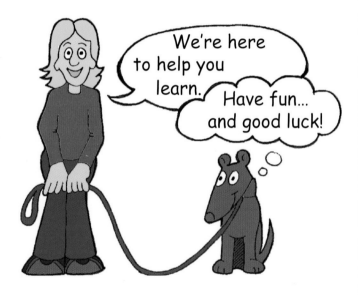

INTRODUCTION TO BASIC TERMINOLOGY

Medical terminology can be a challenge to anyone choosing to enter any field of health care. Learning the **secret codes** to unlock the pronunciation and meaning of medical terminology can be interesting and fun at the same time. Allow your sense of humor free reign to help with the learning process. So, let's work together and learn the language of medical terminology, which is rooted in ancient Greek and Latin.

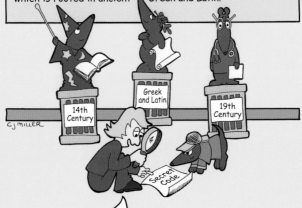

Medical terminology takes a subject or a **word root** and makes a story or explanation by adding information about the word root through the use of a **suffix** or **prefix** and a **combining vowel** to tie the term together. We, in the health care profession, must be able to understand and properly use this terminology. Let's begin to learn how to master the rules of building medical terms.

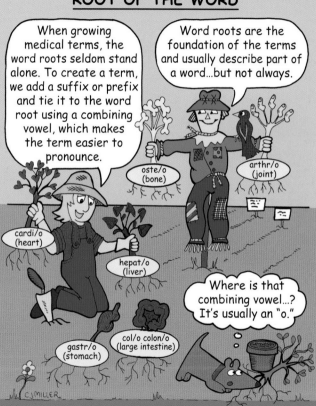

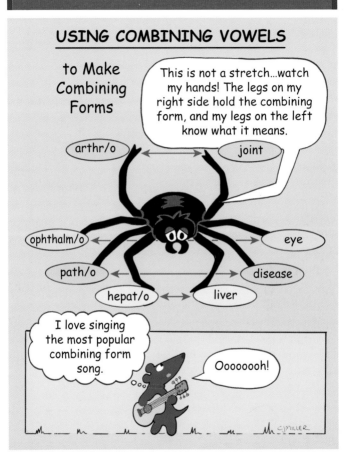

SUFFIX—IT'S AT THE END OF THE WORD

You know the suffixes always follow the word root.

Give meaning to the suffixes— four darts for a dollar!

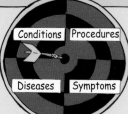

Conditions | Procedures
Diseases | Symptoms

They also complete the term by changing the meaning to "pertaining to" or "abnormal conditions."

Hey...easy on my end with those suffixes.

-pathy
-megaly
-algia
-scopy
(Suffix examples)

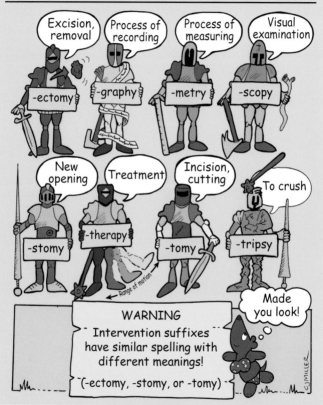

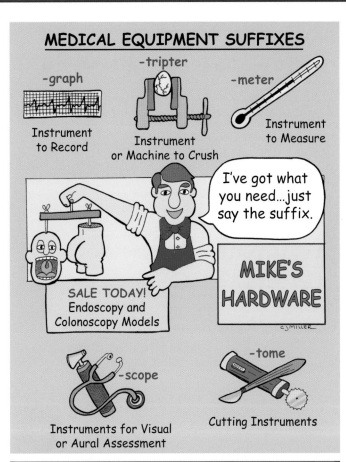

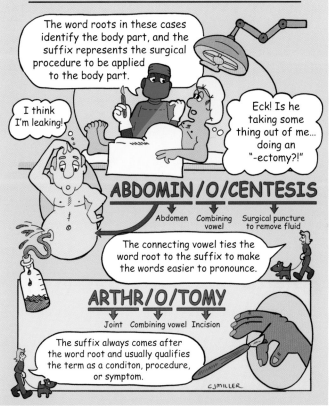

SUFFIXES AND SURGICAL ISSUES

The word roots in these cases identify the body part, and the suffix represents the surgical procedure to be applied to the body part.

I think I'm leaking!

Eck! Is he taking some thing out of me... doing an "-ectomy?!"

ABDOMIN /O/ CENTESIS

Abdomen   Combining vowel   Surgical puncture to remove fluid

The connecting vowel ties the word root to the suffix to make the words easier to pronounce.

ARTHR /O/ TOMY

Joint   Combining vowel   Incision

The suffix always comes after the word root and usually qualifies the term as a conditon, procedure, or symptom.

CJMILLER

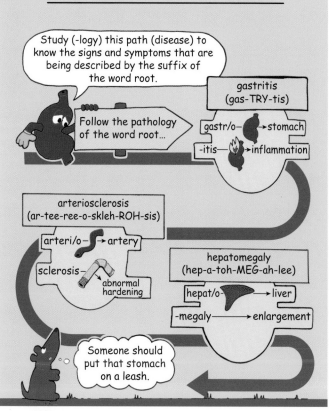

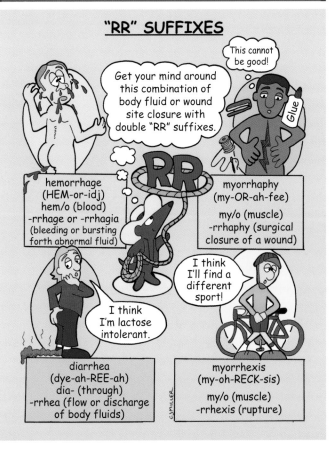

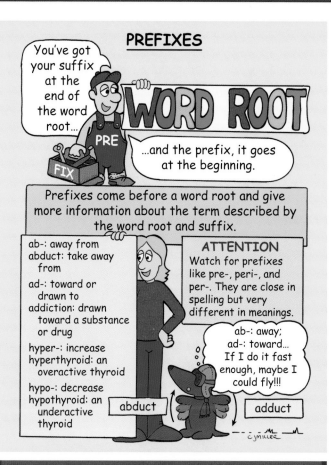

RULES FOR USING SINGULAR AND PLURAL FORMS

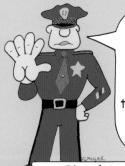

STOP! LOOK!
Pronounce these words. Remember that most medical terms end in Latin or Greek suffixes. Making them plural or singular is not always done the same way as it is done in English.

Singular	Plural
vertebra (VUR-tuh-brah)	vertebrae (VUR-tuh-bray)
diagnosis (dye-agg-NOH-sis)	diagnoses (dye-agg-NOH-seez)
phalanx (FAY-lanks)	phalanges (fuh-LAN-jeez)
bacterium (back-TEER-ree-um)	bacteria (back-TEER-ree-uh)
digitus (DIJ-ih-tus)	digiti (DIJ-ih-tye)
therapy (THAIR-ah-pee)	therapies (THAIR-ah-peez)

GUIDELINES TO FORMING UNUSUAL PLURAL FORMS

When I show up at the end of a word, I usually make the word singular, as in the word "vertebra." If you want the word to be plural, drop me off and add my friend "ae."

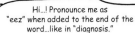

Yep...I make the word plural. I'm pronounced like a long sound of "a," "e," or "i," depending on the term being described, as in "vertebrae."

I make the word singular, as in "diagnosis," when I'm at the end of the term. To make it plural, drop "is" and add "es."

Hi...! Pronounce me as "eez" when added to the end of the word...like in "diagnosis."

When I show up at the end of the term, I usually make it singular, as in the word "phalanx" (oh, that means finger or toe...). To make it plural, drop the "nx" and add "nges."

I sound like a combination of the sound "ng," as in "sing," and the ending "jeez," making the term plural, as in "phalanges."

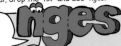

I'm "um." I make words like "bacteria" singular. So, if you drop me and add my friend "a," it becomes plural, as in "bacteria." Cool, huh?

I'm "us," as in the word "digitus." To make me plural, add an "i," and pronounce me as "eye," as in "digiti."

When I'm at the end of the word, I'm pronounced as an "e," like in the word "therapy."

I make "y" plural, which sounds like "eez," as in the word "therapies."

CJMILLER

ANATOMICAL, POSITIONAL, AND DIRECTIONAL TERMS

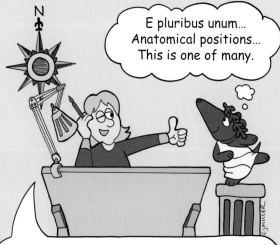

> E pluribus unum... Anatomical positions... This is one of many.

You caught me at my drawing table. At times we may need to describe or explain a location or area of the external or internal body in positional and directional terms. Traditional English terms cannot be used appropriately. Terms of Latin or Greek orgin have been historically used to describe anatomical positions and directional terms.

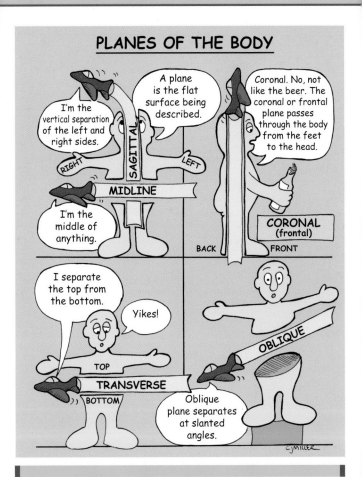

VERTICAL PLANE

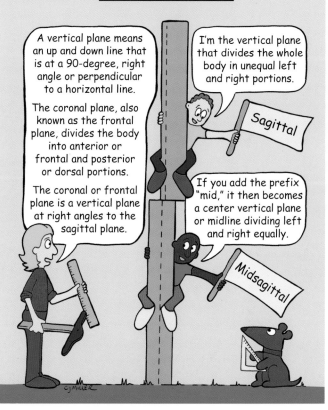

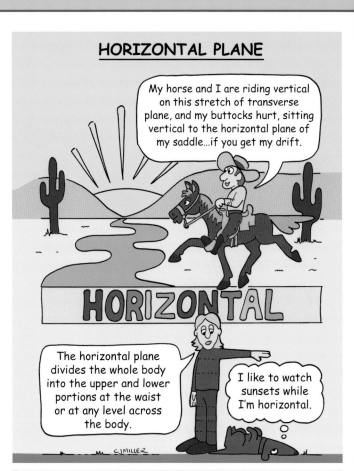

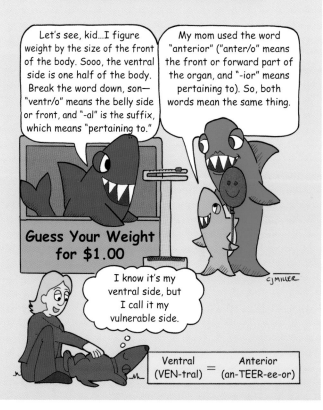

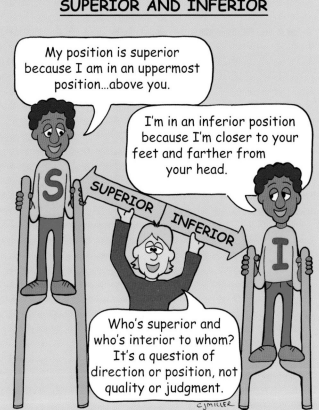

CEPHALIC AND CAUDAL

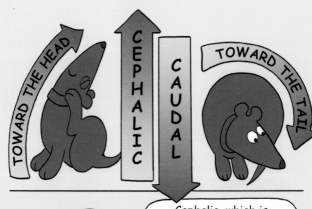

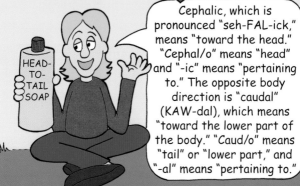

Cephalic, which is pronounced "seh-FAL-ick," means "toward the head." "Cephal/o" means "head" and "-ic" means "pertaining to." The opposite body direction is "caudal" (KAW-dal), which means "toward the lower part of the body." "Caud/o" means "tail" or "lower part," and "-al" means "pertaining to."

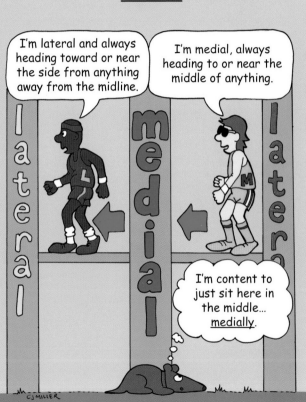

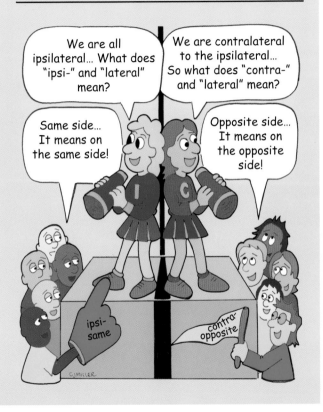

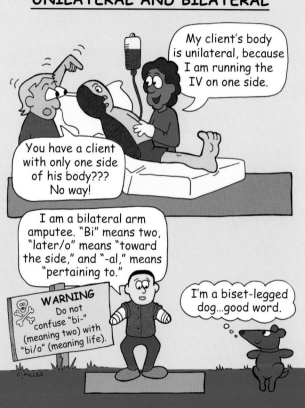

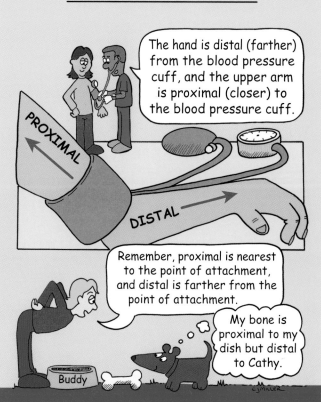

PROXIMAL AND DISTAL

The hand is distal (farther) from the blood pressure cuff, and the upper arm is proximal (closer) to the blood pressure cuff.

PROXIMAL

DISTAL

Remember, proximal is nearest to the point of attachment, and distal is farther from the point of attachment.

My bone is proximal to my dish but distal to Cathy.

Buddy

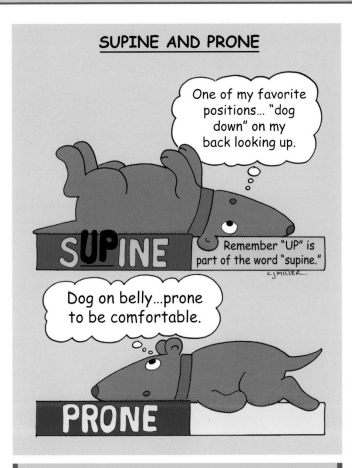

SUPINATE AND PRONATE

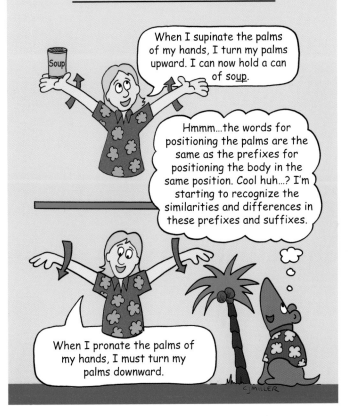

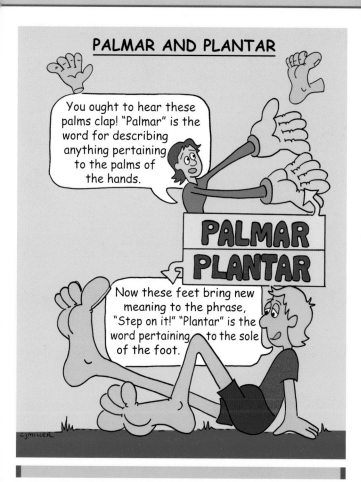

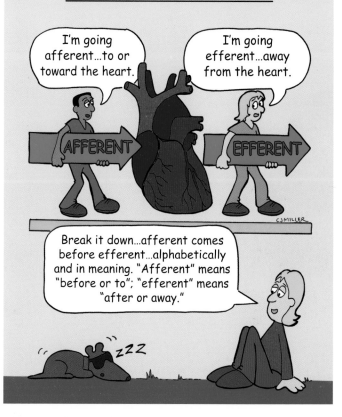

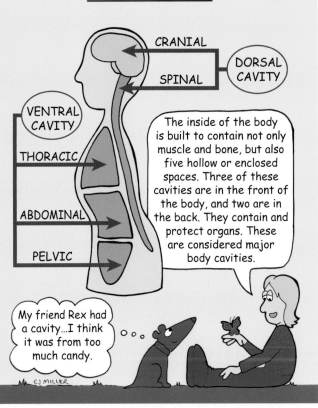

BODY CAVITIES

CRANIAL

SPINAL

DORSAL CAVITY

VENTRAL CAVITY

THORACIC

ABDOMINAL

PELVIC

The inside of the body is built to contain not only muscle and bone, but also five hollow or enclosed spaces. Three of these cavities are in the front of the body, and two are in the back. They contain and protect organs. These are considered major body cavities.

My friend Rex had a cavity...I think it was from too much candy.

CJ MILLER

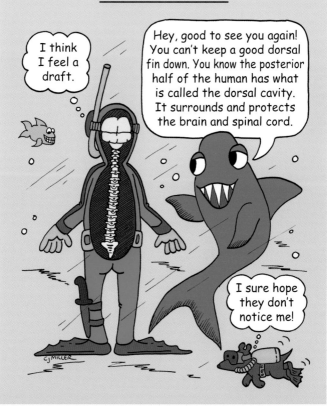

CRANIAL AND SPINAL CAVITIES

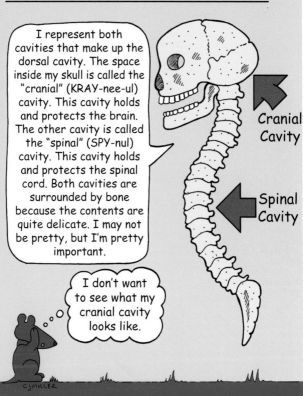

I represent both cavities that make up the dorsal cavity. The space inside my skull is called the "cranial" (KRAY-nee-ul) cavity. This cavity holds and protects the brain. The other cavity is called the "spinal" (SPY-nul) cavity. This cavity holds and protects the spinal cord. Both cavities are surrounded by bone because the contents are quite delicate. I may not be pretty, but I'm pretty important.

I don't want to see what my cranial cavity looks like.

Cranial Cavity

Spinal Cavity

VENTRAL CAVITY

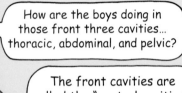

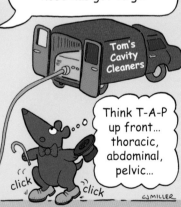

THORACIC CAVITY

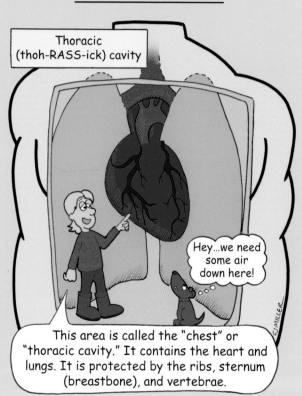

Thoracic
(thoh-RASS-ick) cavity

Hey...we need
some air
down here!

This area is called the "chest" or
"thoracic cavity." It contains the heart and
lungs. It is protected by the ribs, sternum
(breastbone), and vertebrae.

ABDOMINAL AND PELVIC CAVITIES

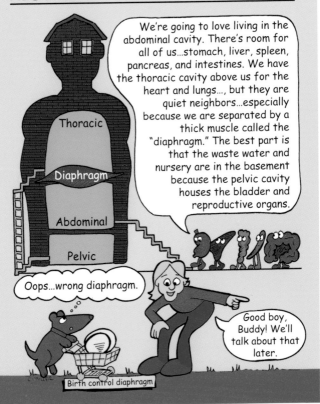

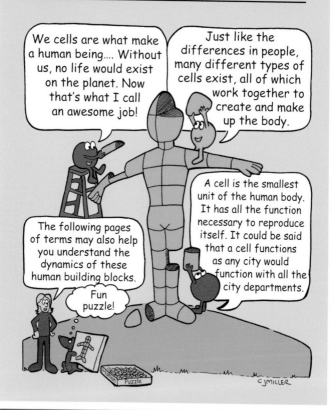

CYTOLOGY

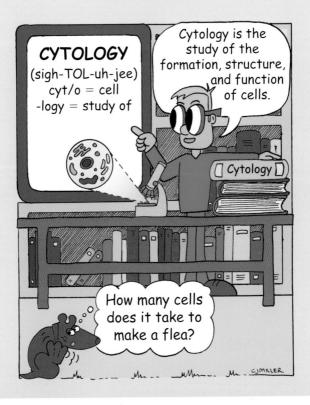

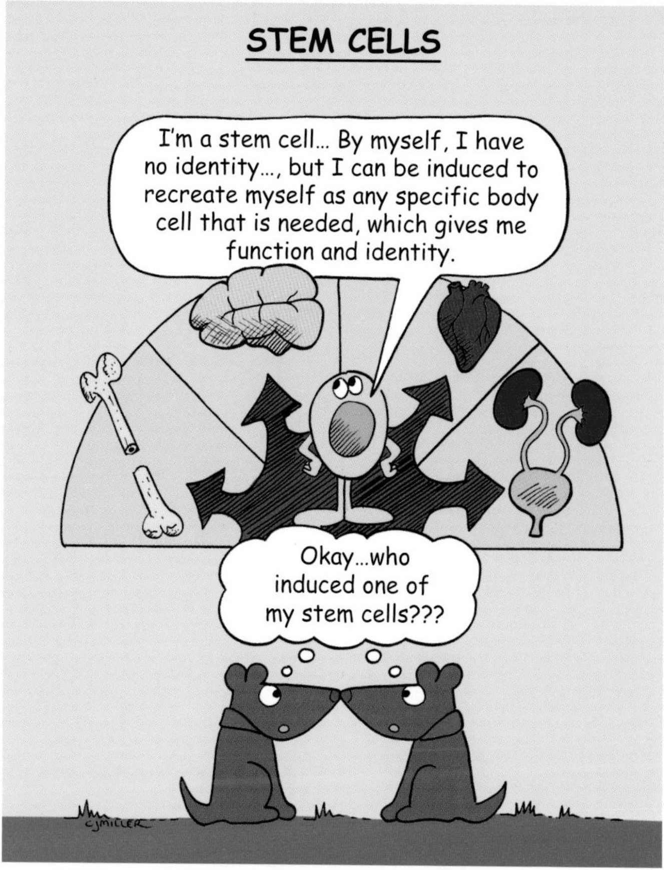
STEM CELLS
I'm a stem cell... By myself, I have no identity..., but I can be induced to recreate myself as any specific body cell that is needed, which gives me function and identity.
Okay...who induced one of my stem cells???
CJMILLER

SOURCES OF STEM CELLS

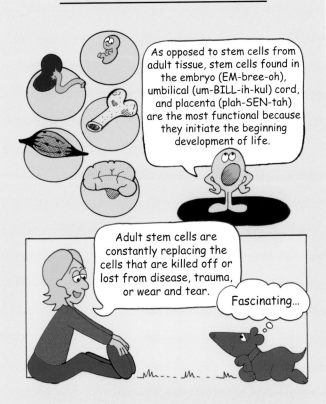

CELL MEMBRANE

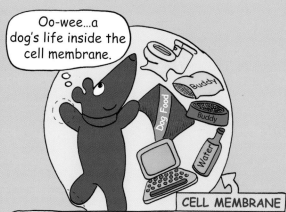

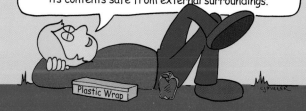

CYTOPLASM

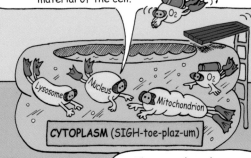

Hi...! Nucleus here. That's the mitochondrion over there...and oxygen molecules coming and going. We all live together in this pool of cytoplasm. "Cyt/o" means "cell" and "-plasm" means "formative material of the cell."

Lysosome

Nucleus

Mitochondrion

O₂

O₂

CYTOPLASM (SIGH-toe-plaz-um)

CJMILLER

How do we get out of this cell?

The cytoplasm has a liquid density that keeps the membrane (MEM-brain) inflated and able to hold its shape while allowing oxygen and nutrients to pass through the wall to support and protect the cell parts (organelles).

NUCLEUS

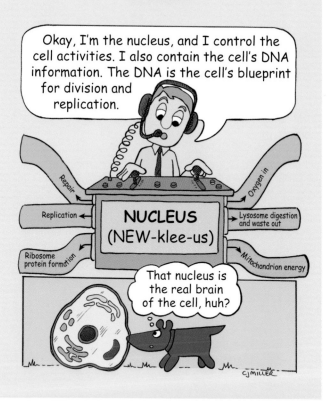

CHROMOSOMES

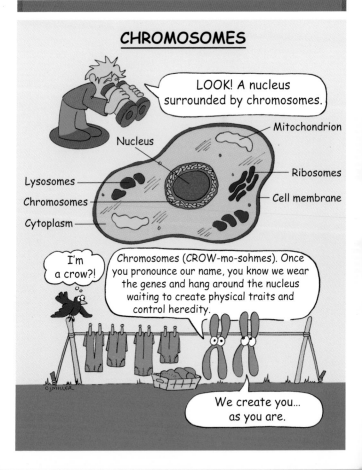

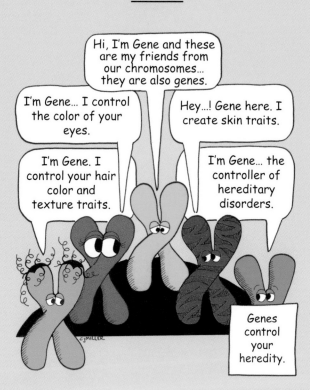

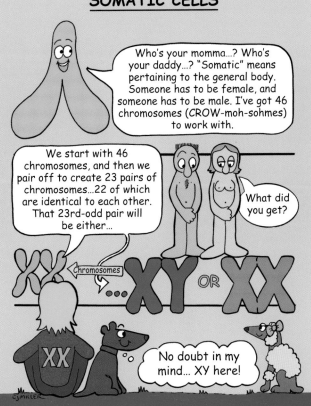

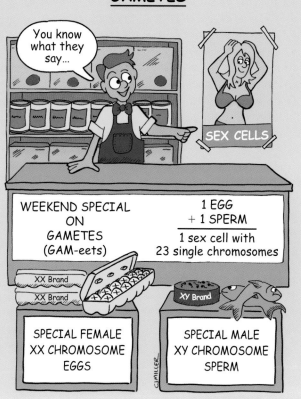

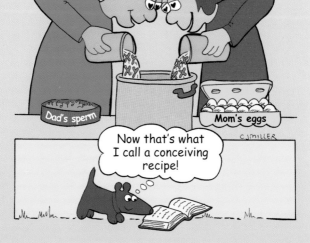

DNA

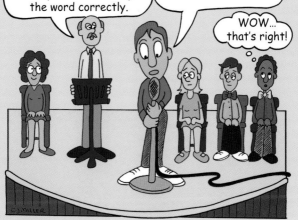

GENOME

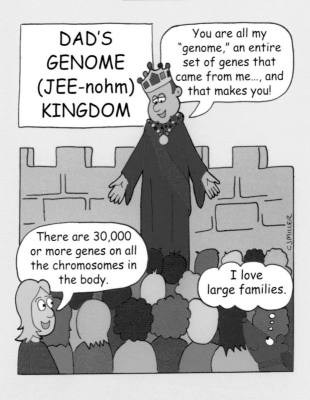

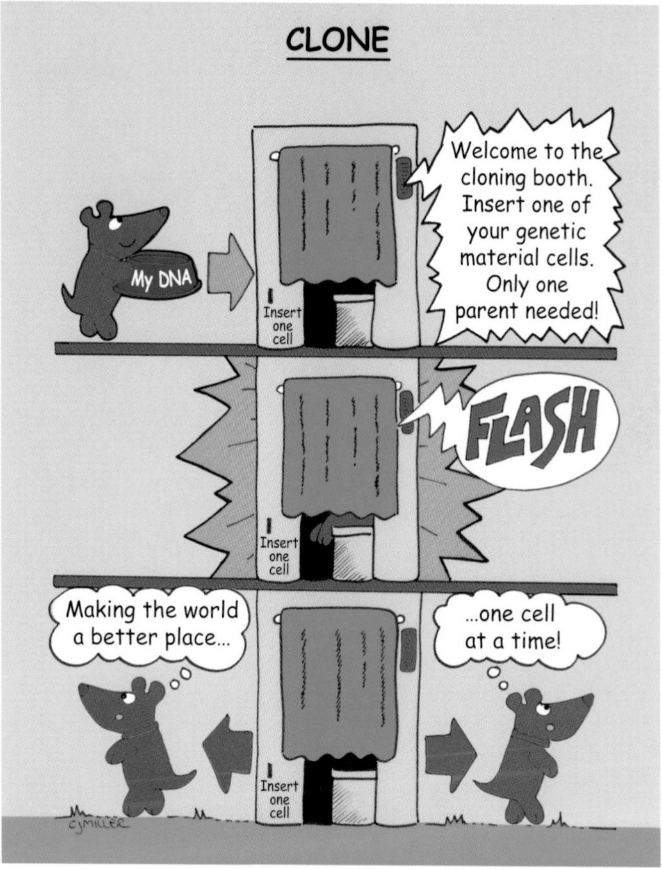
CLONE
My DNA
Welcome to the cloning booth. Insert one of your genetic material cells. Only one parent needed!
Insert one cell
FLASH
Insert one cell
Making the world a better place...
...one cell at a time!
Insert one cell
CJMILLER

TISSUE

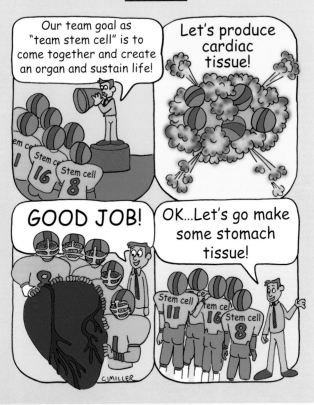

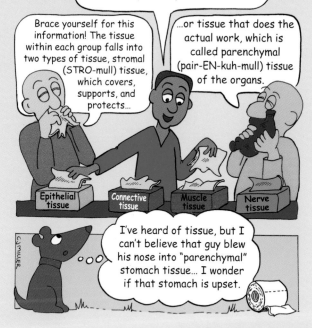

EPITHELIAL TISSUE

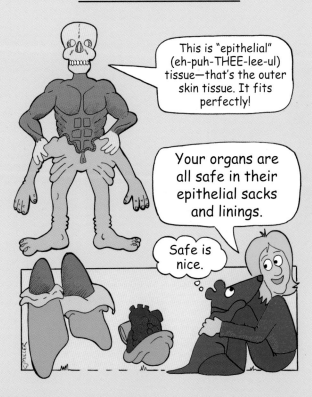

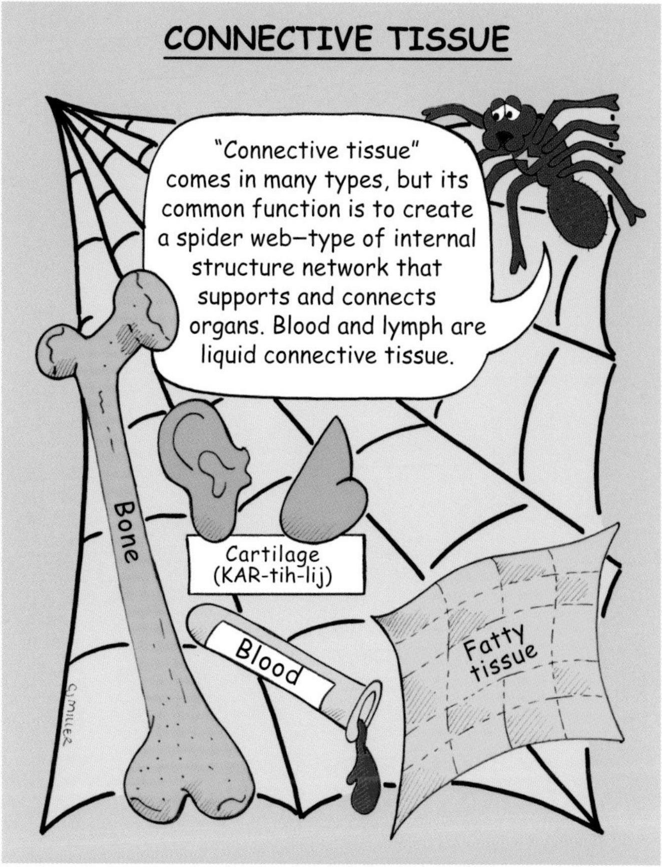
CONNECTIVE TISSUE
"Connective tissue" comes in many types, but its common function is to create a spider web–type of internal structure network that supports and connects organs. Blood and lymph are liquid connective tissue.
Bone
Cartilage (KAR-tih-lij)
Blood
Fatty tissue

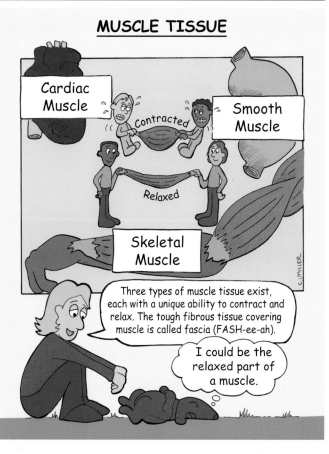

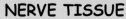

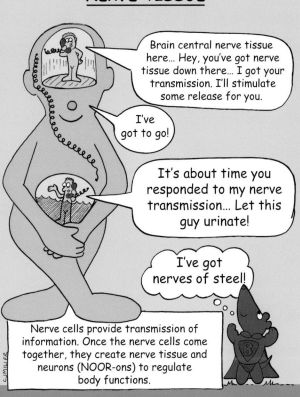

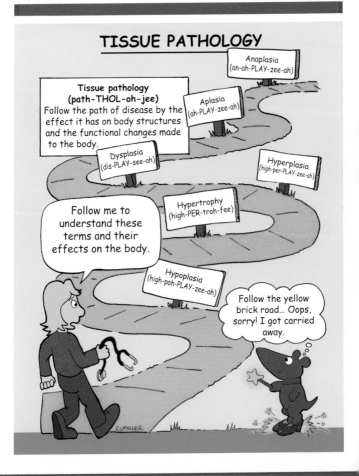

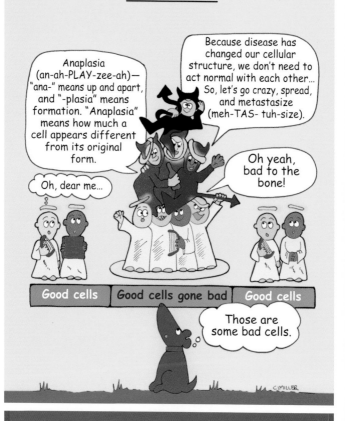

APLASIA

Aplasia (ah-PLAY-zee-ah)
When cells don't form correctly

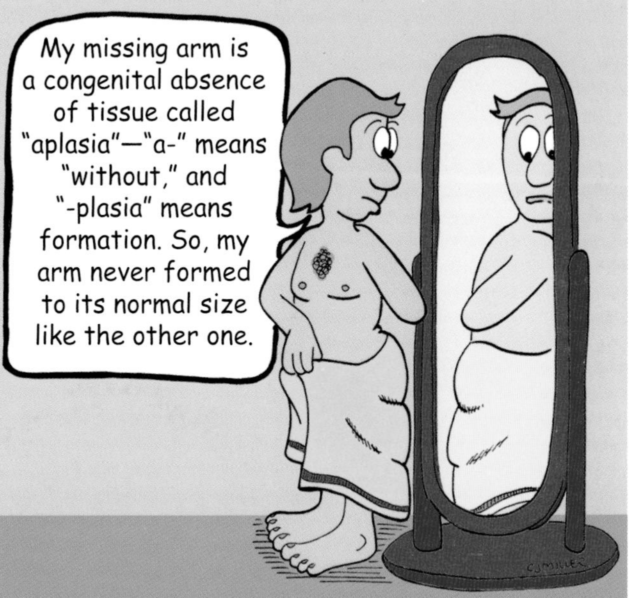

DYSPLASIA

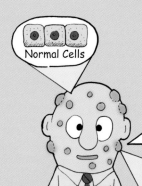

Normal Cells

Yep, these ugly bumps... it's like something in my body got mad at my face. I guess that's why they call these abnormal growths dysplasia (dis-PLAY-zee-ah) with "dys-," meaning "bad," and "-plasia," meaning formation.

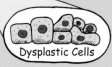

Dysplastic Cells

The body is such an amazing organism, but a "pathogen" can create "dysplasia," interrupting the body's natural development and appearance.

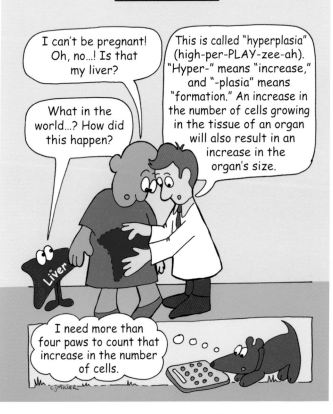

HYPERTROPHY

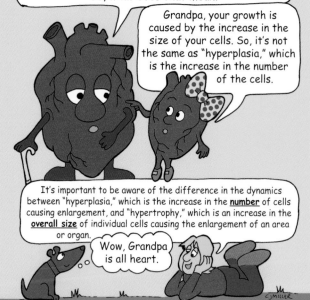

Bigger is not always better! Look at me, I have hypertrophy (high-PER-troh-fee). "Hyper-" means "excessive," and "-trophy" means "development." So, what does that mean?

Grandpa, your growth is caused by the increase in the size of your cells. So, it's not the same as "hyperplasia," which is the increase in the number of the cells.

It's important to be aware of the difference in the dynamics between "hyperplasia," which is the increase in the **number** of cells causing enlargement, and "hypertrophy," which is an increase in the **overall size** of individual cells causing the enlargement of an area or organ.

Wow, Grandpa is all heart.

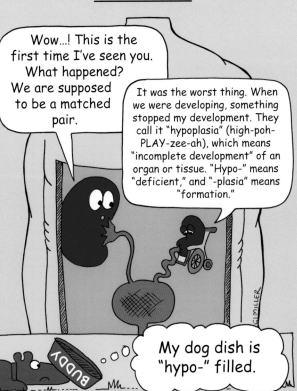

CONGENITAL DISORDERS

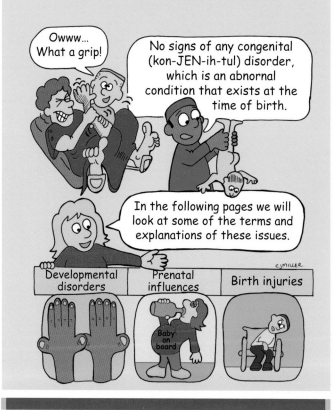

ANOMALY

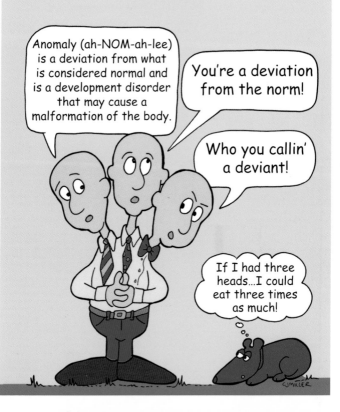

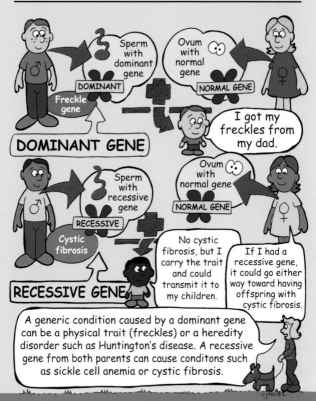

GENETIC DISORDERS

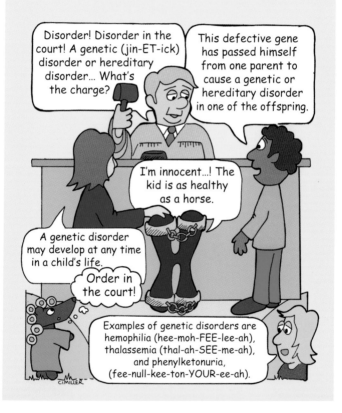

Disorder! Disorder in the court! A genetic (jin-ET-ick) disorder or hereditary disorder... What's the charge?

This defective gene has passed himself from one parent to cause a genetic or hereditary disorder in one of the offspring.

I'm innocent...! The kid is as healthy as a horse.

A genetic disorder may develop at any time in a child's life.

Order in the court!

Examples of genetic disorders are hemophilia (hee-moh-FEE-lee-ah), thalassemia (thal-ah-SEE-me-ah), and phenylketonuria, (fee-null-kee-ton-YOUR-ee-ah).

CIMILLER

CYSTIC FIBROSIS

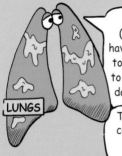

Oh, no-o-o! It's cystic fibrosis (sis-tic figh-BROH-sis)! My lungs have thick mucus that make it difficult to breathe. Bacteria and viruses love to grow in it, causing infection, tissue damage, and, in severe cases, death.

This stuff has me so clogged up. I can't release digestive enzymes, so I need to take enzymes and vitamin supplements.

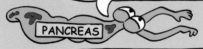

A defective recessive gene transmitted from the parents causes cystic fibrosis. Respiratory and digestive symptoms show up early in infancy.

This stuff with defective genes is very scary.

DOWN SYNDROME
DOWN'S SYNDROME

Preferred spelling

 TRISOMY **21** (DEFECTIVE GENE)

CREATES A SYNDROME
(SIN-drohm) or group
of signs and symptoms

**WITH VARYING DEGREES OF
MENTAL RETARDATION**

**MULTIPLE PHYSICAL
ABNORMALITIES**

HEMOPHILIA

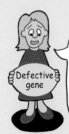

Hemophilia (hee-moh-FILL-ee-ah) is a hereditary bleeding disorder caused by a defective gene that I passed down to my son. It's typically transmitted from mother to son.

Defective gene

I have a missing clotting factor that won't allow my blood to clot... not good. I bleed from my nose, gums, ears, rectum, and any skin scrape or laceration. I also have problems with edema and joint swelling as a result of the bleeding.

I have hemophilia—a product of one of my mother's defective genes.

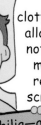

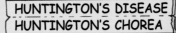

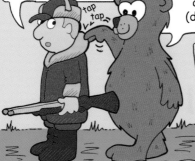

MUSCULAR DYSTROPHY

Muscular dystrophy (DIS-troh-fee) is a gene-transmitted disease that causes progressive weakness and deterioration of muscle tissue.

What's amazing is that muscular dystrophy consists of 20 or more inherited muscle weakness disorders, but it doesn't affect the nervous system.

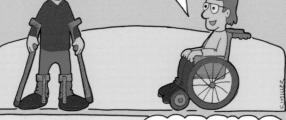

Duchenne's (doo-SHENZ) muscular dystrophy affects only males. Symptoms appear between 2 and 6 years of age.

Could this be muscular dissatisfaction?

PHENYLKETONURIA

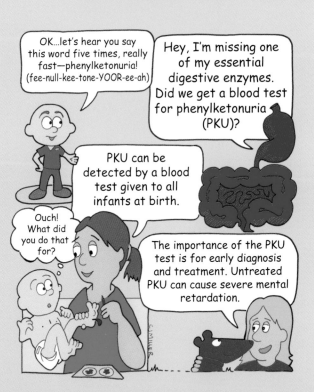

SICKLE CELL ANEMIA

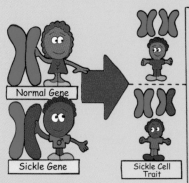

Sickle cell anemia is the most common hereditary disorder among African Americans. The disease is only expressed in offspring who inherit the gene from both parents. If only one gene is present, the off-spring will have the sickle cell trait but not the disease.

The defective gene causes abnormal hemoglobin (HEE-moh-gloh-bin) to create red blood cells with sickle shapes. The sickle-shaped red blood cells cannot bend and therefore block the flow of blood leading to clumping, blockage, and ischemia (is-KEE-mee-ah), which is oxygen-deprived tissue.

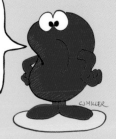

TAY-SACHS DISEASE

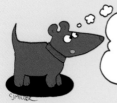

Who names these diseases? Was it someone named "Tay" with the last name "Sachs," or was it two people... "Tay" and "Sachs?"

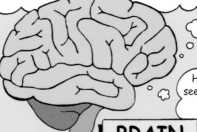

Tay-Sachs (TAY-sacks) disease is an inherited disease caused by the transmission of a defective gene. It occurs in individuals of Eastern-European Jewish origin and is caused by a deficiency of an enzyme, leading to central nervous system (CNS) deterioration and early death.

Has anyone seen my missing enzyme?

BRAIN

-LOGIST AND -LOGY

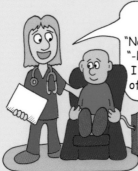

I'm a nephrologist (neh-FRAH-luh-jist). "Nephr/o" means "kidneys" and "-logist" means "specialist." I specialize in the treatment of diseases of the kidneys.

DIALYSIS (die-AL-us-sis)

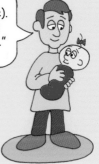

My field of medical study is neonatology (nee-oh-nay-TALL-uh-gee). "Neo-" means "new," "nat/o" means "birth," and "-logy" means "study of." I specialize in newborns.

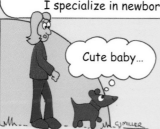

Cute baby...

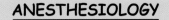

ANESTHESIOLOGY

CARDIOLOGY

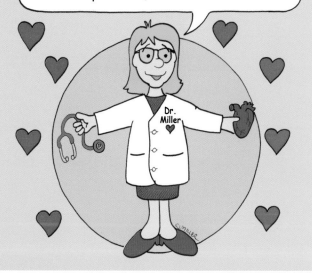

When I went through school, I specialized in cardiology (kar-dee-ALL-uh-jee). "Cardi/o" means "heart," and "-logy" means the "study of." So I became a cardiologist (kar-dee-ALL-uh-jist). The suffix, "-ist," means "specialist," and I love what I do!

DERMATOLOGY

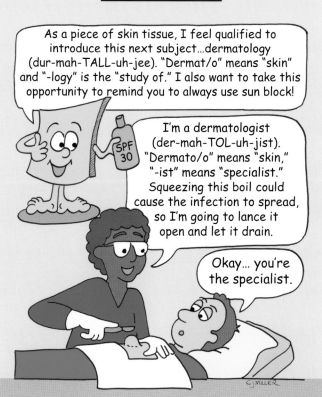

As a piece of skin tissue, I feel qualified to introduce this next subject...dermatology (dur-mah-TALL-uh-jee). "Dermat/o" means "skin" and "-logy" is the "study of." I also want to take this opportunity to remind you to always use sun block!

I'm a dermatologist (der-mah-TOL-uh-jist). "Dermato/o" means "skin," "-ist" means "specialist." Squeezing this boil could cause the infection to spread, so I'm going to lance it open and let it drain.

Okay... you're the specialist.

GERIATRICS

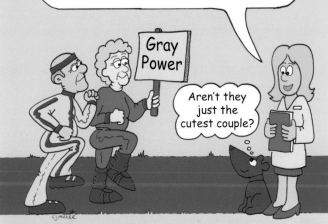

Geriatrics (jair-ee-AT-tricks) is the branch of medicine dealing with the aged. "Ger/o" means "aging," "iatr/o" means "treatment," and "-ics" means "pertaining to." As a geratrician (jair-ee-ah-TRIH-shun), I specialize in the diagnosis and treatment of medical problems of the aging population.

Gray Power

Aren't they just the cutest couple?

GYNECOLOGY

The study of the female body, including the female reproductive system, is called "gynecology" (gye-nuh-KALL-uh-jee). "Gynec/o" means "female," and "-logy" means the "study of." A gynecologist (gye-nuh-KALL-luh-jist) is a specialist in this field.

Wow, studying women! That could be a good gig!

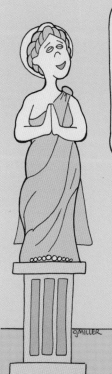

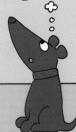

HEMATOLOGY

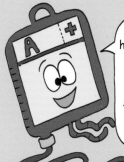

I'm a bag of blood, and I'm here to tell you about hematology (he-mah-TALL-uh-jee). "Hemat/o" means "blood" and "-logy" means the "study of." So, hematology is the medical field that studies and treats me—blood.

A hematologist (he-mah-TALL-luh-jist) is a specialist in the study of blood. A friend of blood is a friend of mine... anytime!

HISTOLOGY

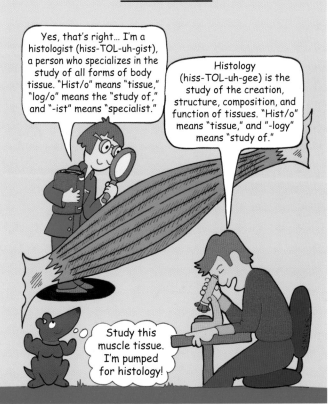

IMMUNOLOGY

Immunology (im-you-NOL-uh-jee) is the study of the reaction of tissues to antigen stimulation. "Immun/o" means "to protect," and "-logy" means the "study of." A specialist in the study of the immune system is an immunologist (im-you-NOL-uh-jist).

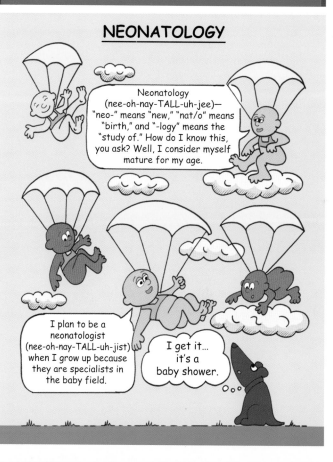

NEUROLOGY

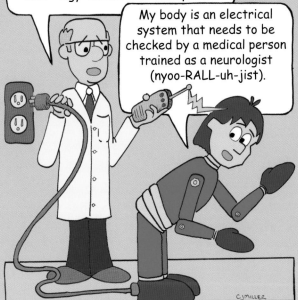

ONCOLOGY

Oncology (on-KALL-uh-jee) is the study and treatment of all tumors with a focus on cancer cells. "Onc/o" means "tumor," and "-logy" means the "study of."

I have a creepy feeling that someone is watching. I bet it's that cancer specialist, the oncologist.

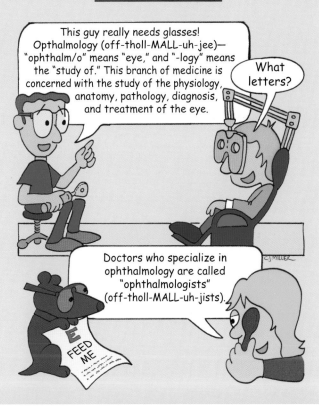

ORTHOPEDICS
AND OTHER RELATED FIELDS

Rheumatoid arthritis (ROO-mah-toyd arth-RYE-tis) is characterized by the inflammation of connective tissue. Specialists in this area who diagnose and treat rheumatic diseases are called "rheumatologists" (roo-ma-TALL-uh-jists).

An orthopedist (or-thoh-PEE-dist) specializes in the diagnosis and treatment of bone, joint, and muscle problems.

Orthotics (or-THOT-ics) is the making and fitting of special braces and splints to support, align, or correct deformities and function of movable body parts.

Podiatry (po-DIE-a-tree) is the specialized care of the feet by podiatrists (po-DIE-uh-trists). "Pod/o" means "foot," and "-iatrist" means one who specializes in treatment.

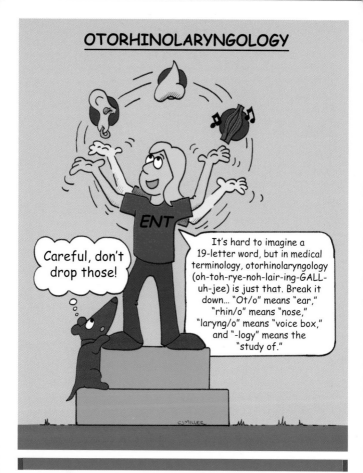

PATHOLOGY

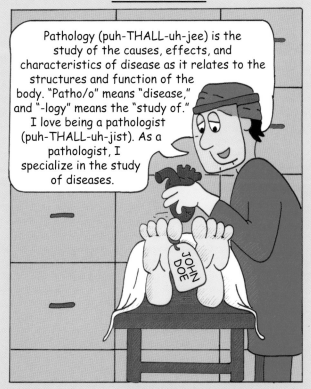

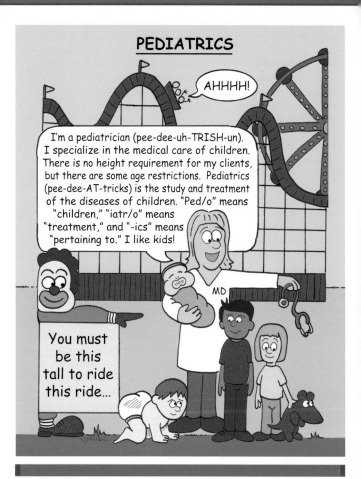

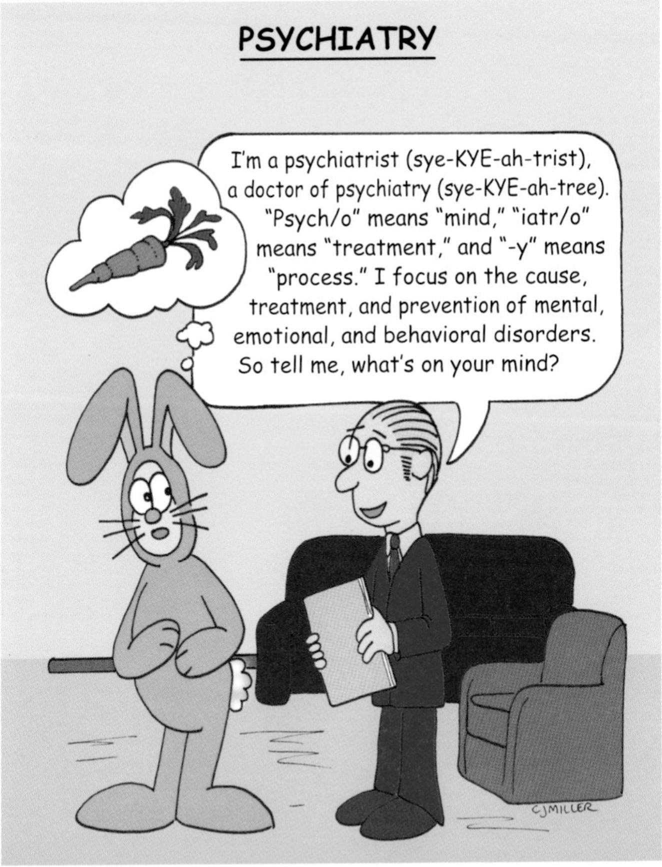
PSYCHIATRY
I'm a psychiatrist (sye-KYE-ah-trist), a doctor of psychiatry (sye-KYE-ah-tree). "Psych/o" means "mind," "iatr/o" means "treatment," and "-y" means "process." I focus on the cause, treatment, and prevention of mental, emotional, and behavioral disorders. So tell me, what's on your mind?
CJMILLER

UROLOGY

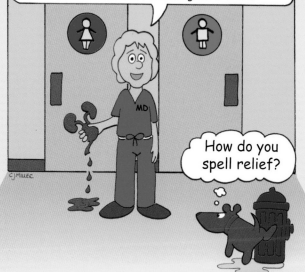

Urology (yoo-RALL-uh-jee) is the study and treatment of diseases of the urinary tract. "Ur/o" means "urinary system," and "-logy" means the "study of." As a urologist (yoo-RALL-uh-jist), I specialize in the field that deals with the anatomy, physiology, disorders, and care of the urinary tract in both sexes and the male genital tract.

How do you spell relief?

BODY SYSTEMS AND MAIN STRUCTURES

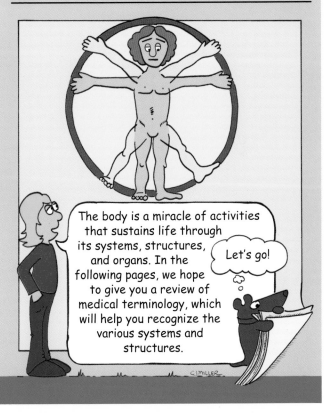

The body is a miracle of activities that sustains life through its systems, structures, and organs. In the following pages, we hope to give you a review of medical terminology, which will help you recognize the various systems and structures.

Let's go!

MUSCULOSKELETAL SYSTEM

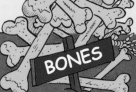

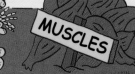

The musculoskeletal (muss-skyoo-loh-SKELL-uh-tul) system is made up of bones, joints, articulations (ar-tick-yoo-LAY-shuns), and muscles. This system works as a framework, protects the organ systems, and provides the body's ability to move.

BONE TISSUE

Hey, I'm in the compact bone and am a second layer called "spongy bone" or "cancellous" (KAN-seh-lus) bone. The medullary cavity and red bone marrow lie within my spongy layer.

Hello...I'm the medullary (MED-you-lehr-ee). I'm located in the shaft of the long bone surrounded by compact bone and filled with yellow bone marrow.

Hi, I'm the endosteum (en-DOS-tee-um). I'm the tissue that forms the lining of the medullary cavity.

Call me periosteum (pehr-ee-OSS-tee-um). "Peri-" means "surrounding," "oste/o" means "bone," and "-um" means "structure" or "thing." I'm the tough outer bone cover of fibrous tissue.

I'm compact bone. I'm hard, dense, and very strong. I form the outer layer of the periosteum.

JOINTS

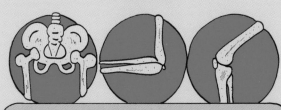

Synovial (sin-NOH-vee-ul) joints are the movable joints of the body. They can be ball-and-socket or hinged joints.

Some joints in the skull are sutures, which means "to stitch," and they are immovable joints. Symphysis (SIM-fih-sis) joints are two bones joined by cartilage (KAR-tih-lij), which are only slightly movable joints.

That's a lot of joints.

CARTILAGE

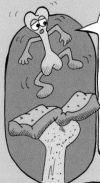

Cartilage (KAR-tih-lij) is the rubbery connective tissue that works as a shock absorber between bone and is more elastic and flexible than bone.

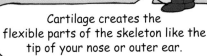

Cartilage creates the flexible parts of the skeleton like the tip of your nose or outer ear.

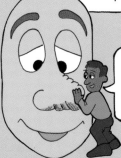

Articular (ar-TICK-you-lar) cartilage covers the ends of many bones and serves a protective function.

MUSCLES

The term "muscle" comes from the Latin, "musculus" or "mus," meaning "mouse." Think of the muscle contracting under the skin as the scurrying of little mice.

- Muscles contract and relax.
- Muscles are attached to bones by tendons.

1. Skeletal muscle assists the body to move.
2. Smooth muscle is responsible for the movement of organs.

3. Cardiac muscle helps pump blood via the circulatory system.

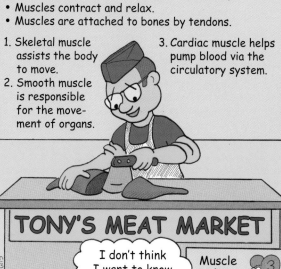

MUSCLE FIBERS AND FASCIA

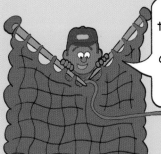

Muscle fibers held together by a fibrous sheath and connective tissue are what compose a muscle.

Connective Tissue

Fascia Muscle Fabrication

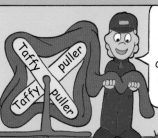

Taffy puller

Taffy puller

I'm here producing fascia (FASH-ee-ah), which is a sheet of tough connective tissue that covers, supports, and separates muscles.

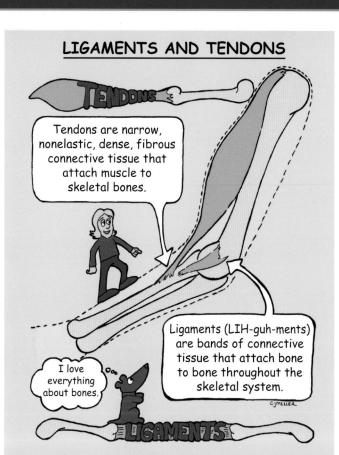

MUSCLE PATHOLOGY

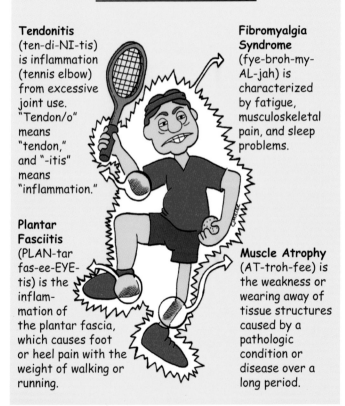

Tendonitis (ten-di-NI-tis) is inflammation (tennis elbow) from excessive joint use. "Tendon/o" means "tendon," and "-itis" means "inflammation."

Fibromyalgia Syndrome (fye-broh-my-AL-jah) is characterized by fatigue, musculoskeletal pain, and sleep problems.

Plantar Fasciitis (PLAN-tar fas-ee-EYE-tis) is the inflammation of the plantar fascia, which causes foot or heel pain with the weight of walking or running.

Muscle Atrophy (AT-troh-fee) is the weakness or wearing away of tissue structures caused by a pathologic condition or disease over a long period.

INTRODUCTION
TO CARDIOVASCULAR TERMS

The superior vena cava, along with other veins, returns waste and deoxygenated blood back from the body tissue.

The aorta and arteries move oxygenated blood away from the heart to be delivered to the tissues of the body.

The heart is part of the cardiovascular (kar-dee-oh-VASS-kyoo-lur) system. "Cardi/o" means "heart," "vascul/o" means "blood vessels," and "-ar" means "pertaining to." The heart is an electrically stimulated muscular pump that continually moves blood products, oxygen, and nutrients to body tissue while removing cellular waste.

Let's take a tour of the heart and its related structures.

The Heart

ARTERIES

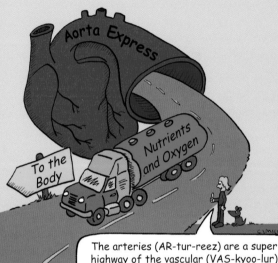

The arteries (AR-tur-reez) are a super highway of the vascular (VAS-kyoo-lur) system. Just like our freeways, the arteries are bigger and thicker. They expand and contract with each pressurized beat of the heart. The arteries move fluid and blood products with enough pressure to carry nutrients and oxygenated blood to support even the most distal body tissue.

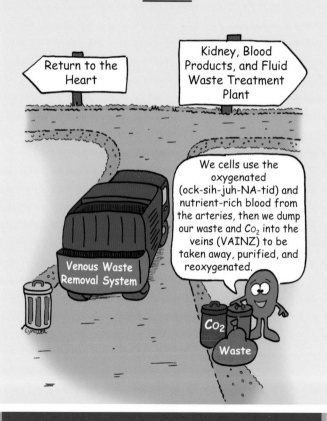

BLOOD CELL TYPES AND COMPONENTS

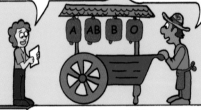

I see your red blood cells have the A, B, or AB antigens (AN-tih-juns) and the O type with no antigen. I need three units of O+...stat!

Yes, I can get all four major blood types for you... A, AB, B, and O! I will get O+ typed and crossed for you.

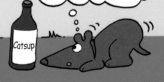

Typing and crossmatching ensures patients receive blood that is compatible with their own to prevent a transfusion reaction, which can be serious and life threatening.

Red stuff on a hot dog...? That makes me nervous.

Catsup

EXTRAVASATION

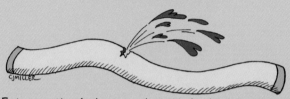

Extravasation (ecks-trav-ah-SAY-shun) is a term that means the process of a substance (blood and lymph) leaking outside the vessel into surrounding tissue. "Extra-" means "outside," "vas/o" means "vessel," and "-ation" means the "process of." Examples would be...

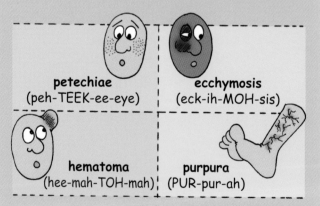

petechiae
(peh-TEEK-ee-eye)

ecchymosis
(eck-ih-MOH-sis)

hematoma
(hee-mah-TOH-mah)

purpura
(PUR-pur-ah)

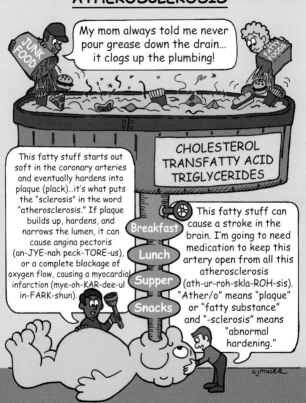

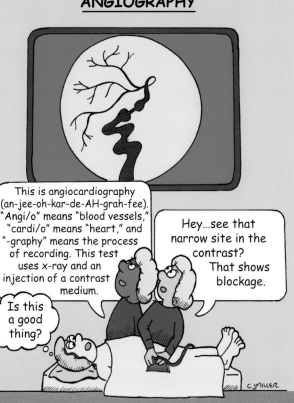

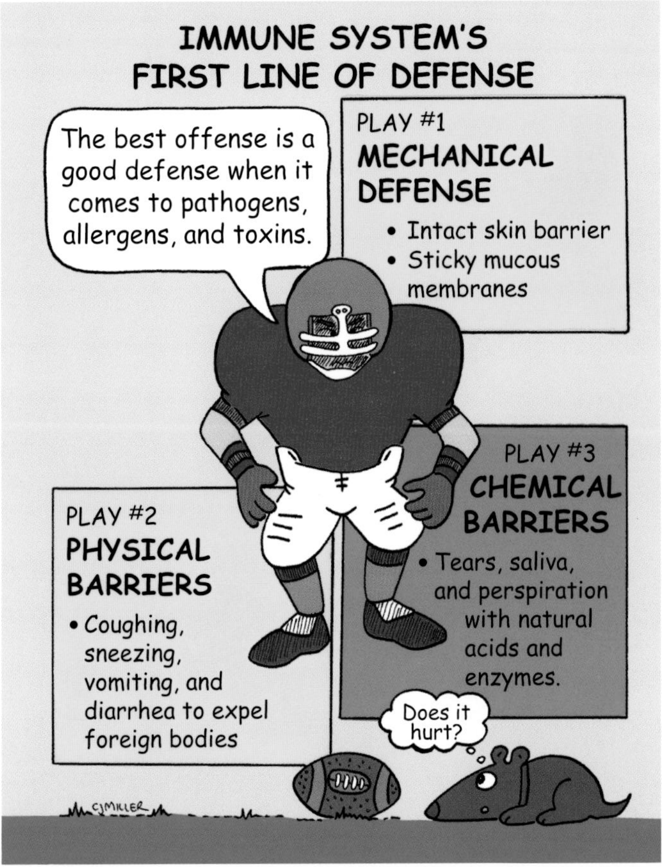
IMMUNE SYSTEM'S FIRST LINE OF DEFENSE
The best offense is a good defense when it comes to pathogens, allergens, and toxins.
PLAY #1
MECHANICAL DEFENSE
• Intact skin barrier
• Sticky mucous membranes
PLAY #2
PHYSICAL BARRIERS
• Coughing, sneezing, vomiting, and diarrhea to expel foreign bodies
PLAY #3
CHEMICAL BARRIERS
• Tears, saliva, and perspiration with natural acids and enzymes.
Does it hurt?
CJMILLER

IMMUNE SYSTEM'S SECOND LINE OF DEFENSE

If pathogens get past the first line of defense, they enter the bloodstream and are consumed by neutrophils and monocytes, a process called **phagocytosis** (fag-oh-sye-TOH-sis).

Inflammation is a protective response to injury that causes heat, swelling, redness, and pain, which in turn causes vasoconstriction and increased vascular permeability. If caused by a pathogen, the inflammation is called an infection.

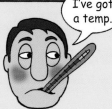

I've got a temp.

Pyrexia (py-RECK-see-uh) is a fever that serves to increase the action of phagocytes and to decrease the viability of some pathogens.

IMMUNE SYSTEM'S THIRD LINE OF DEFENSE

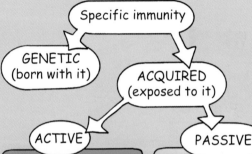

Specific immunity

GENETIC (born with it)

ACQUIRED (exposed to it)

ACTIVE

PASSIVE

NATURAL—Development of memory cells from second exposure

ARTIFICIAL— Vaccination or immunization

NATURAL—Passage of antibodies through placenta or breast milk

ARTIFICIAL—Use of immunoglobins harvested from a donor

Antibodies that make up your specific immune system are called **immunoglobulins** (ih-myoo-noh-GLOB-you-lins).

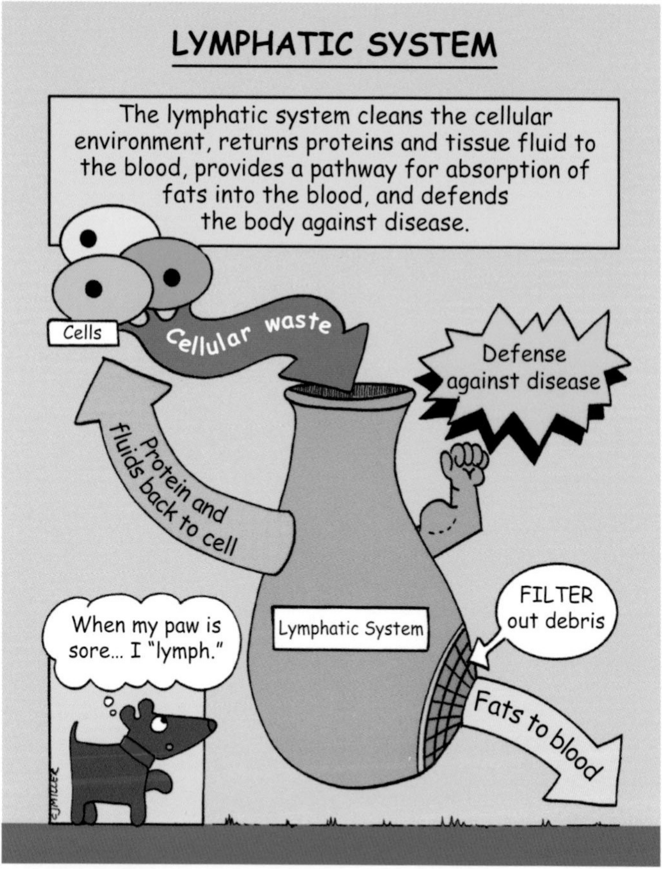
LYMPHATIC SYSTEM
The lymphatic system cleans the cellular environment, returns proteins and tissue fluid to the blood, provides a pathway for absorption of fats into the blood, and defends the body against disease.
Cells
Cellular waste
Defense against disease
Protein and fluids back to cell
Lymphatic System
FILTER out debris
When my paw is sore... I "lymph."
Fats to blood
EJMILLER

LYMPH VESSELS

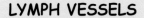

Cervical lymph gland

Thymus gland

Axillary lymph node

Spleen

Inguinal lymph node

Right lymphatic duct

The right side of the head, neck, and upper quadrant of the body drain into the right lymphatic duct, which drains to the right subclavian vein.

Thoracic duct

The remaining areas of the body drain into the thoracic duct, which returns lymph fluid back into the blood system by emptying into the left subclavian vein.

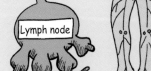

Lymph node

Popliteal lymph node

Lacteals (LACK-tee-ahls) are the capillaries in the villi in the walls of the small intestine. They absorb fat and fat-soluble vitamins and carry them into the bloodstream.

If you were a "lymphduck," would that make you a lame duck?

SMILLER

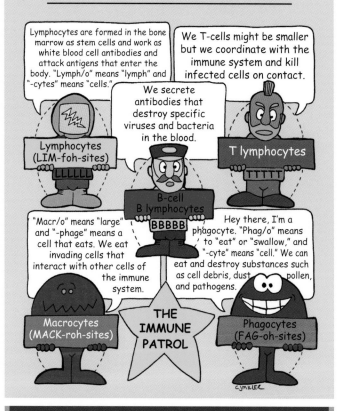

SPLEEN

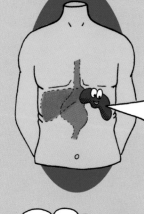

I'm the spleen. You can find me perched in the left upper quadrant of the abdomen—just inferior to the diaphragm and posterior to the stomach. I'm the part of the lymphatic system that filters the blood, destroys worn-out red blood cells, and produces special white blood cells that support the immune system.

How spleen-did.

CJMILLER

RESPIRATORY SYSTEM

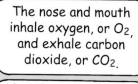

The nose and mouth inhale oxygen, or O_2, and exhale carbon dioxide, or CO_2.

The voice box, or larynx, (LAIR-inks) is within the respiratory system. When we exhale, our vocal cords vibrate to produce sound, but if we stop to inhale and take a breath, we have to stop talking.

The lungs are able to remove CO_2, which is carried in the venous deoxygenated blood.

CJMILLER

The respiratory (ress-pir-ah-TOR-ee) system has the important job of bringing oxygen-rich air to the body to be delivered to blood cells and distributed to tissues of the body.

NOSE AND PHARYNX

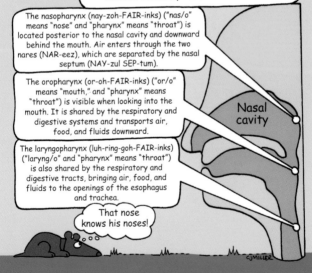

Welcome to the nasal cavity (NAY-zul KAV-it-ee)! It's an area lined with specialized tissue called the "mucous membrane." This membrane secretes mucus to protect and lubricate. The olfactory (ol-FACK-toh-ree) nerve endings are located in the upper part of the nasal cavity, giving you your sense of taste and smell. As we travel deeper into this cavity, you will find the pharynx (FAIR-inks), which is commonly known as the "throat."

The nasopharynx (nay-zoh-FAIR-inks) ("nas/o" means "nose" and "pharynx" means "throat") is located posterior to the nasal cavity and downward behind the mouth. Air enters through the two nares (NAR-eez), which are separated by the nasal septum (NAY-zul SEP-tum).

The oropharynx (or-oh-FAIR-inks) ("or/o" means "mouth," and "pharynx" means "throat") is visible when looking into the mouth. It is shared by the respiratory and digestive systems and transports air, food, and fluids downward.

The laryngopharynx (luh-ring-goh-FAIR-inks) ("laryng/o" and "pharynx" means "throat") is also shared by the respiratory and digestive tracts, bringing air, food, and fluids to the openings of the esophagus and trachea.

Nasal cavity

That nose knows his noses!

CJMILLER

STRUCTURES OF THE LUNGS

The trachea (TRAY-kee-ah) is the airway into the lungs and is also known as the "windpipe."

The bronchial tree is separated into branches called "bronchi" (BRONG-kye). One bronchus goes into each lung, where it branches into smaller bronchioles (BRONG-kee-ohls).

Alveoli (al-VEE-oh-lye) are grapelike clusters known as air sacs located at the end of each bronchiole.

The lungs are divided into lobes. The right lung has three lobes—one on top of the other. The left lung has two lobes and is slightly smaller than the right.

The beauty of the various parts of the respiratory (RESS-pur-ah-tore-ee) system is that they can be compared with an upside-down tree. The root system of any tree must be directed to its life source, which for the bronchial tree is up and out of the body to access the oxygen that surrounds us. The bronchial tree ends in what looks like leaf buds, the alveoli.

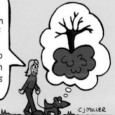

CJ MILLER

TONSILS

I think you are stepping on my gag reflex!

We are the tonsils. Sitting at the base of the tongue are the lingual (LING-gwal) tonsils. "Lingual" means "pertaining to the tongue." Sitting next to us on both sides are the palatine (PAL-ah-tyne) tonsils. "Palatine" means "referring to the hard and soft palates."

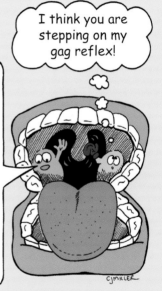

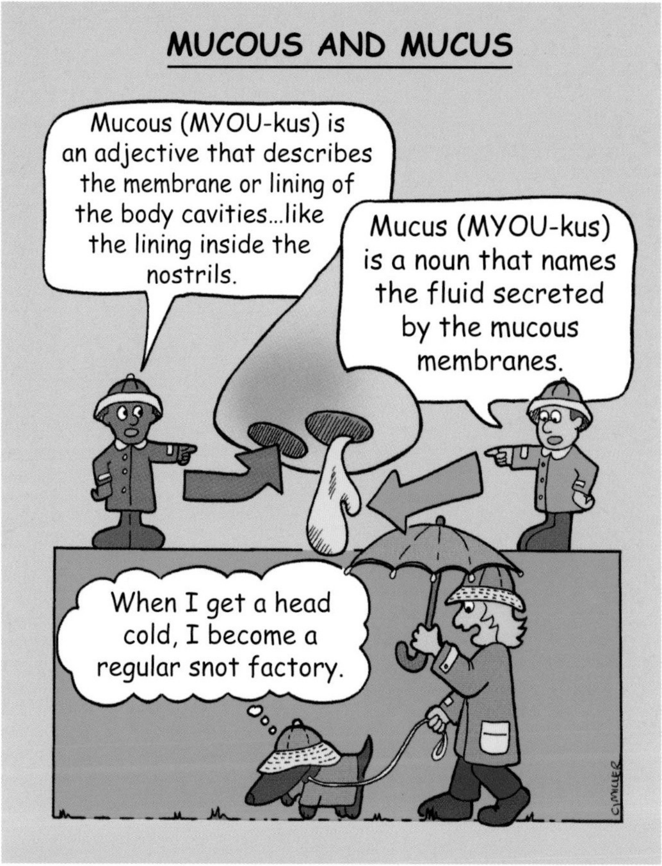
MUCOUS AND MUCUS
Mucous (MYOU-kus) is an adjective that describes the membrane or lining of the body cavities...like the lining inside the nostrils.
Mucus (MYOU-kus) is a noun that names the fluid secreted by the mucous membranes.
When I get a head cold, I become a regular snot factory.
CJMILLER

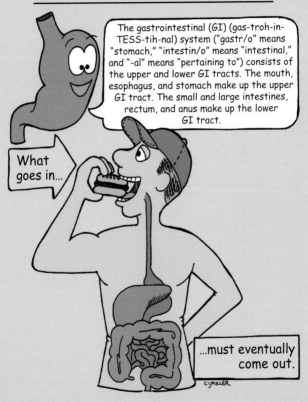

MOUTH, ESOPHAGUS, AND STOMACH

Helloooo, I am the mouth or oral cavity. I am made up of many parts. I have lips; two palates (PAL-ats)—one hard palate and one soft palate—that form the roof of my mouth; and a strong flexible muscle called the tongue, which gets quite a workout when I talk, chew, or swallow food. My teeth or dentition (den-TISH-un) are the naturally arranged teeth in my maxillary (upper) and mandibular (lower) arches.

Oral Cavity

Esophagus

I'm the esophagus (eh-SOF-uh-gus). I'm a flexible tube that leads from the pharynx of the mouth to the stomach and the lower esophageal sphincter or cardiac sphincter (SFINK-ter).

The stomach is a saclike organ composed of the fundus (upper rounded part); the body (main portion); the antrum (lower part); and the pyloric (pyle-LOR-ick) sphincter, the ringlike muscle that controls the flow from the stomach to the small intestine.

Stomach

Call it tripe or call it menudo... it's still stomach to me.

C.J.MILLER

ABDOMEN AND STOMACH

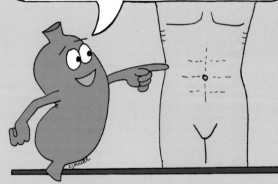

The word "abdomen" (AB-do-min) refers to a "region"...and "stomach" (STOM-ick) refers to an "organ."

The combining form "gastr/o" refers only to the "stomach" (the organ), whereas the combining forms "abdomin/o," "lapar/o," and "celi/o" refer to the "abdomen" (region).

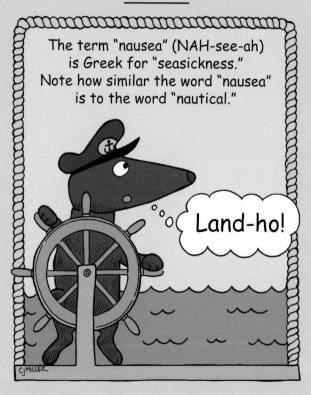

SMALL AND LARGE INTESTINE

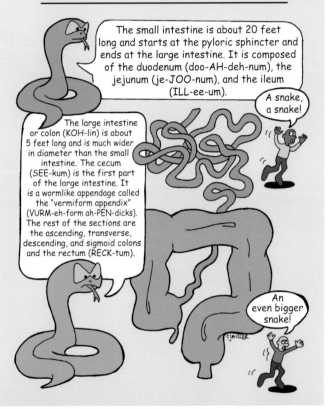

The small intestine is about 20 feet long and starts at the pyloric sphincter and ends at the large intestine. It is composed of the duodenum (doo-AH-deh-num), the jejunum (je-JOO-num), and the ileum (ILL-ee-um).

A snake, a snake!

The large intestine or colon (KOH-lin) is about 5 feet long and is much wider in diameter than the small intestine. The cecum (SEE-kum) is the first part of the large intestine. It is a wormlike appendage called the "vermiform appendix" (VURM-eh-form ah-PEN-dicks). The rest of the sections are the ascending, transverse, descending, and sigmoid colons and the rectum (RECK-tum).

An even bigger snake!

LIVER, PANCREAS, AND GALLBLADDER

I'm the liver. I filter out toxins from the blood and turn food into fuel and nutrients. The term "hepatic" (heh-PAT-ick) means "pertaining to the liver" ("hepat/o" means "liver," and "-ic" means "pertaining to").

I'm the pancreas (PAN-kree-us). I have two important functions—one being the secretion of pancreatic juice through the pancreatic duct into the common bile duct and the other an endocrine function controlling blood sugar levels in the body.

Hey, I'm the gallbladder. If I'm inflamed, I have cholecystitis (koh-lee-sis-TI-tis). "Cholecyst/o" means "gallbladder," and "-itis" means "inflammation." I'm a small sac underneath the right lobe of the liver, and I I store bile.

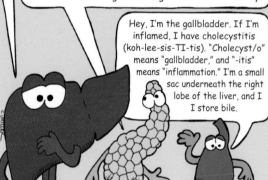

URINARY SYSTEM

The urinary system or urinary tract consists of two kidneys, two ureters, one bladder, and one urethra.

Keeping a balance or homeostasis (hoh-mee-oh-STAY-sis) in our system is very important. "Home/o" means "sameness," and "-stasis" means "control." The urinary tract keeps balance among water, salts, and acids. It also reabsorbs water as needed to keep the body in a homeostasis or balanced state.

Hey…you two kidneys! Will you slow the flow down a bit? If this guy doesn't pee soon, I'm going to blow up!

The urinary system removes waste material, regulates fluid volume, and maintains electrolyte concentration.

Excuse me… this will just take a second.

KIDNEYS, URETERS, URINARY BLADDER, PROSTATE, AND URETHRA

We are the kidneys. "Renal" (REE-nal) means "pertaining to the kidneys." We are the dialysis unit for the body, filtering the blood as it constantly moves through our nephrons. The waste products and toxins are removed and sent to the renal pelvis to be released from the body.

We are the two ureters (YOOR-eh-turs), which are 10- to 12-inch tubes that move urine by peristalsis (pair-ih-STALL-sis) from the kidneys to the bladder. We don't do anything too exciting, but every once in a while, we might get blocked by a renal stone... Oooh, ouch, those hurt!

I'm the urinary bladder. Call me the reservoir for the urine. I can expand and extract. Usually I carry about a pint of urine in my grapefruit-sized hollow muscular organ.

I'm the prostate. Though I'm not part of the urinary system, my placement can raise havoc in males when I become enlarged and constrict the urethra. The bladder has a hard time emptying then.

I'm the urethra (yoo-REE-thrah). I come in two sizes...long (male) and short (female). I'm the one-way exit of urine from the body. I have two flow-control sphincters—one at the drain area of the bladder and the other at the meatus (mee-ATE-us) (the body's exit point). Remember, the words "ureter" and "urethra" are very close in sound and spelling.

-URIA AND UREA

These two words look alike..., but they aren't the same. "Urea" refers to the "chemical waste product" excreted by the kidneys.

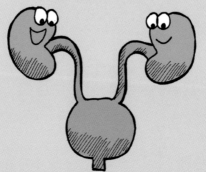

"-Uria" is a suffix that means "urinary condition," such as in the word "pyuria" (pye-YOOR-ee-ah), which means "pus in the urine." "Py/o" means "pus," and "-uria" means a "urinary condition."

NERVOUS SYSTEM

The nervous system consists of the central nervous system (CNS), which includes the brain and spinal cord, and the peripheral nervous system (PNS), which consists of nerves that extend from the brain and spinal cord to the tissues of the body.

The CNS is our body's information highway of stimulus and response. The CNS is the center that coordinates and controls all of the body's activities via the nerves, spinal cord, and sensory organs.

Specialized nerve cells called "interneurons" (in-tur-NOOR-ons) make the connection between sensory and motor neurons.

Stimulus response! See cat...want to chase it!

SPINAL CORD

The spinal cord starts at the medulla oblongata (muh-DOO-lah ob-lon-GAH-tah) and ends at a structure called the "cauda equina" (KAH-dah eh-KWY-nah), which means "horse's tail."

The cord is protected from damage by vertebrae (vur-ta-bray) and a tissue insulation called the "meninges" (meh-NIN-jeez).

Looks like a centipede with a big head.

STRUCTURES OF THE BRAIN

The thalamus (THAL-uh-mus) is located below the cerebrum, and it produces sensation by relaying impulses from the cerebrum and the sense organs of the body.

The cerebrum (suh-REE-brum) is the largest and uppermost portion of the brain. It's responsible for thought, judgment, memory, and emotion.

The hypothalamus (HYE-poh-thal-ah-mus) is responsible for regulating seven major body functions. "Hypo" means "below," so the hypothalamus is located below the thalamus.

The brainstem is the connection between the cerebral hemispheres and the spinal cord and consists of the midbrain, pons, and medulla (muh-DOO-lah). Injure this stem and the game is over.

EYE

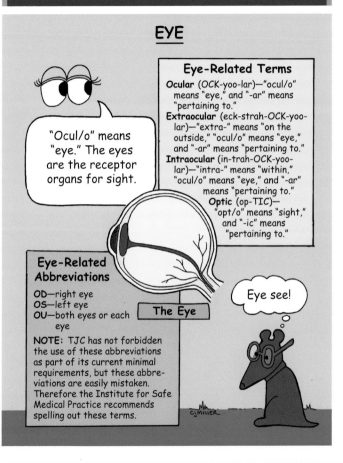

Eye-Related Terms

Ocular (OCK-yoo-lar)—"ocul/o" means "eye," and "-ar" means "pertaining to."

Extraocular (eck-strah-OCK-yoo-lar)—"extra-" means "on the outside," "ocul/o" means "eye," and "-ar" means "pertaining to."

Intraocular (in-trah-OCK-yoo-lar)—"intra-" means "within," "ocul/o" means "eye," and "-ar" means "pertaining to."

Optic (op-TIC)— "opt/o" means "sight," and "-ic" means "pertaining to."

"Ocul/o" means "eye." The eyes are the receptor organs for sight.

Eye-Related Abbreviations

OD—right eye
OS—left eye
OU—both eyes or each eye

NOTE: TJC has not forbidden the use of these abbreviations as part of its current minimal requirements, but these abbreviations are easily mistaken. Therefore the Institute for Safe Medical Practice recommends spelling out these terms.

The Eye

Eye see!

CORE/O AND CORNE/O

"Core/o" means "pupil of the eye."
A corectome (kor-RECK-tome) would
be an instrument used to
cut the pupil.

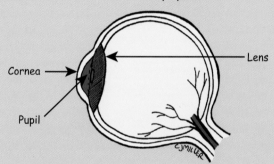

Cornea

Pupil

Lens

"Corne/o" means "cornea," the clear,
transparent covering of the eye. "Corneal"
means "pertaining to the cornea."
Corneitis (kor-neeh-EYE-tis) is an
inflammation (-itis) of the cornea.

EAR

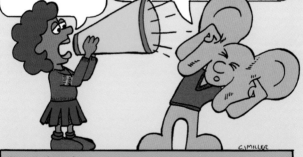

"Auris" is Latin for "ear." The function of the ear is to receive sound impulses and transmit them to the brain! The inner ear maintains our body's balance!

Not so loud! I can hear you! My auditory (AH-dih-tor-ee) canal is working just fine. "Audi/o" means "hearing," and "-ory" means "pertaining to." The "acoustics" (ah-KOOS-ticks), which mean being "related to sound," are fine. "Acous/o" means "hearing" or "sound," and "-tic" means "pertaining to."

Ear-Related Abbreviations

AD—right ear
AS—left ear
AU—both ears

NOTE: TJC has not forbidden the use of these abbreviations as part of its current minimal requirements, but these abbreviations are easily mistaken. Therefore the Institute for Safe Medical Practice recommends spelling out these terms.

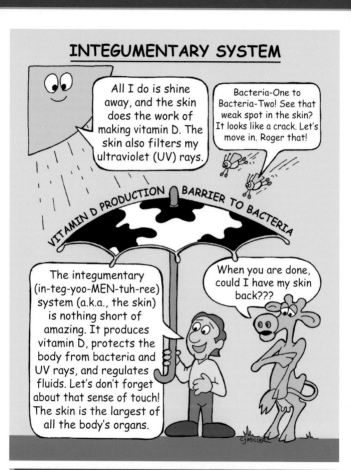

SKIN

Approximately 2 yards of skin cover all external surfaces of the average adult's body. The terms "derm/o," "dermat/o," and "cutane/o" (kyoo-TAY-nee-o), mean "skin." Skin usually fits over our body like a glove, but because of my recent weight loss, my skin is more like a rug.

Skin Layers

Epidermis (ep-ih-DER-mis) Layer

Dermis (DER-mis) Layer

Subcutaneous (sub-kyoo-TAY-nee-us) Layer

ASSOCIATED STRUCTURES OF THE INTEGUMENTARY SYSTEM

Sweat glands, also known as "sudoriferous" (soo-dur-IF-uh-rus) glands, are the body's natural cooling system and assist in waste removal. Body odor associated with sweating comes between perspiration and bacteria on the skin's surface.

Hair follicles are sacs that hold hair fibers. Hair itself is a rodlike structure of tightly fused dead protein cells filled with hard keratin (KAIR-uh-tin).

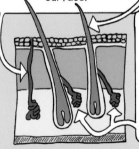

Sebaceous (seh-BAY-shus) glands are located in the dermis (DER-mis) layer and are closely associated with hair follicles. These glands produce sebum (SEE-bum), which lubricates the skin surface and is acidic. These glands interfere with bacterial growth.

Buddy? Did you know that only two places exist on your body that have no hair follicles? That would be the palms of your hands and the soles of your feet.

Some of us are more hairy than others.

CJMILLER

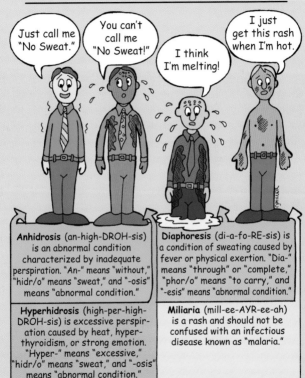

INFECTION AND INFLAMMATION

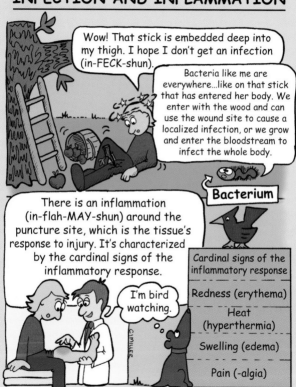

Wow! That stick is embedded deep into my thigh. I hope I don't get an infection (in-FECK-shun).

Bacteria like me are everywhere...like on that stick that has entered her body. We enter with the wood and can use the wound site to cause a localized infection, or we grow and enter the bloodstream to infect the whole body.

Bacterium

There is an inflammation (in-flah-MAY-shun) around the puncture site, which is the tissue's response to injury. It's characterized by the cardinal signs of the inflammatory response.

I'm bird watching.

Cardinal signs of the inflammatory response
Redness (erythema)
Heat (hyperthermia)
Swelling (edema)
Pain (-algia)

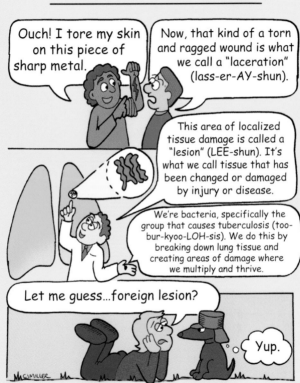

STRATA AND STRIAE

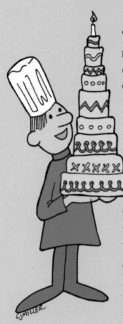

"Strata" means "layers"…like my layer cake or stratum corneum, the outermost layer of the epidermis.

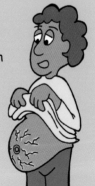

"Striae" means "striped" or "streaked," such as in the term "striation," which is also called "stretch marks."

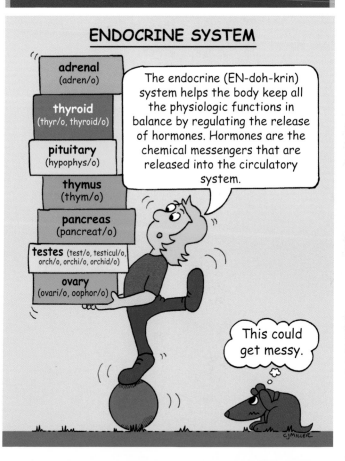

PITUITARY GLAND

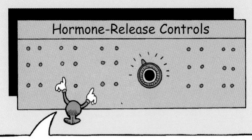

I'm what they call the "master gland." I'm about the size of a pea but large on function. I go by the name of "pituitary" (pih-TOO-ih-tar-ree) gland or "hypophysis" (hye-POFF-ih-sis) gland. My primary function is the secretion of hormones and the control of the other endocrine glands.

Pituitary...that's a fun word to say...pituitary, pituitary.

THYROID GLAND

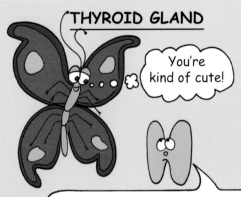

You're kind of cute!

Yikes...I'm the thyroid (THIGH-royd) gland. I'm located in the anterior part of the neck. I regulate the body's metabolism (muh-TAB-boh-lih-sum), as well as normal growth and development. I also regulate the amount of calcium deposited in the bone.

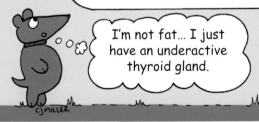

I'm not fat... I just have an underactive thyroid gland.

PARATHYROID GLANDS

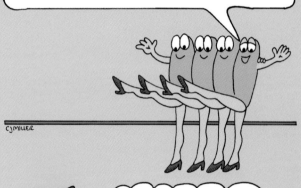

We are the four parathyroid (pair-uh-THIGH-royd) glands. We are located behind the thyroid gland. Although we can't help you dance, we do control the calcium levels in your bones by secreting parathyroid hormone (PTH).

CJMILLER

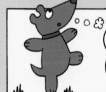

I have a friend named Royd...he thought I should be a dancer. I told him I couldn't because I needed a "pair-of-thighs," Royd.

ADRENAL GLANDS

We are the adrenal (ahh-DREE-nul) glands. We come in pairs, one on top of each kidney... In fact, for that reason, we are sometimes called "suprarenal glands" that make us feel like super heroes or something.

Look inside...we are made up of two separate parts. The adrenal cortex (KORE-tecks) secretes steroids, and the adrenal medulla (muh-DOO-lah) secretes fight-or-flight hormones in times of stress.

Medulla

Cortex

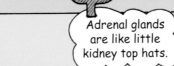

Adrenal glands are like little kidney top hats.

CJMILLER

PANCREAS

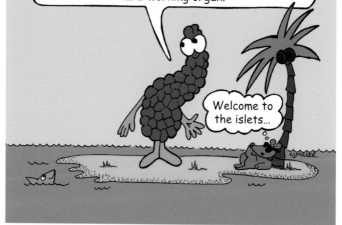

Remember me? I'm the pancreas (PAN-kree-as). I'm also in the gastrointestinal section, but right now, I want to tell you about my endocrine function. Inside me are the pancreatic islets (pan-kree-AT-ick EYE-lets) or the islets of Langerhans (EYE-lets of LANG-ur-hahnz). Those are special endocrine-functioning cells that control blood sugar levels and glucose metabolism. Unlike Buddy, I'm a hard-working organ.

Welcome to the islets...

THYMUS GLAND

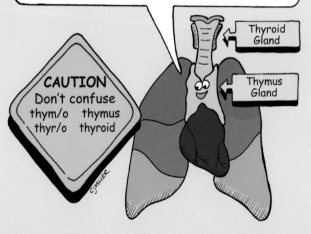

I'm the thymus (THIGH-mus) gland. I'm located in a safe cozy place behind the sternum and above the heart. I'm a lymphoepithelial organ that releases thymosin (THIGH-moh-sin), which stimulates the maturation of lymphocytes into T-cells.

Thyroid Gland

Thymus Gland

CAUTION
Don't confuse
thym/o   thymus
thyr/o   thyroid

TESTES

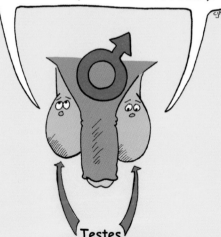

We are the male gonads (GOH-nads), specifically known as the "testes" (TESS-teez), which are part of the male reproductive system. We are responsible for the gametes (GAM-eets) known as "sperm" and for the production of the male hormone, testosterone (tess-TAHS-teh-rohn).

Testes

OVARIES

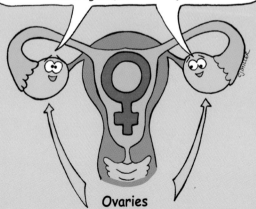

We are the female gonads (GOH-nads), known as the "ovaries" (OH-ver-ees). We are part of the female reproductive system responsible for the storage of a lifetime supply of reproductive gamete (GAM-eet) cells called "ova" or "eggs." We dutifully release ova (approximately one per month) from puberty to menopause. We are also a good source for the production of the female hormone, estrogen (ESS-troh-jin).

Ovaries

MENSTRUAL DISORDERS

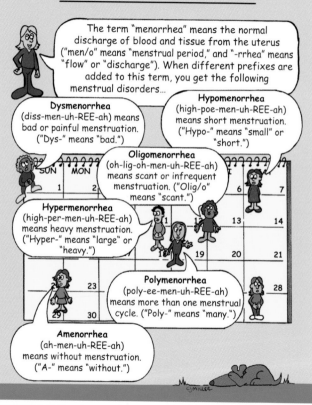

The term "menorrhea" means the normal discharge of blood and tissue from the uterus ("men/o" means "menstrual period," and "-rrhea" means "flow" or "discharge"). When different prefixes are added to this term, you get the following menstrual disorders...

Dysmenorrhea (diss-men-uh-REE-ah) means bad or painful menstruation. ("Dys-" means "bad.")

Hypomenorrhea (high-poe-men-uh-REE-ah) means short menstruation. ("Hypo-" means "small" or "short.")

Oligomenorrhea (oh-lig-oh-men-uh-REE-ah) means scant or infrequent menstruation. ("Olig/o" means "scant.")

Hypermenorrhea (high-per-men-uh-REE-ah) means heavy menstruation. ("Hyper-" means "large" or "heavy.")

Polymenorrhea (poly-ee-men-uh-REE-ah) means more than one menstrual cycle. ("Poly-" means "many.")

Amenorrhea (ah-men-uh-REE-ah) means without menstruation. ("A-" means "without.")

ABNORMAL UTERINE BLEEDING

Well, I certainly don't need "light" protection for my menstrual flow!

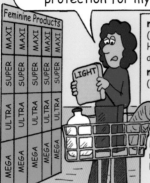

menometrorrhagia
(men-oh-meh-tro-RAH-zsa)
Heavy uterine bleeding during and between menstral periods.

menorrhagia
(men-or-RAH-zsa)
  Heavy or prolonged mentrual flow; may indicate fibroids.

metrorrhagia
  (meh-tro-RAH-zsa)
Bleeding between regular menses; remember the "t" for between. May indicate lesions.

These uterine bleeding terms all mean heavy or excessive vaginal bleeding. The difference is the relationship to the menstrual cycle.

Don't confuse... "-metry" means "the process of measuring," and "metr/o" means "uterus."

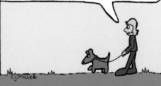

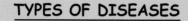

TYPES OF DISEASES

We're ready to introduce some diseases and disorders. We thought we would suit up to keep from catching anything in the process.

They say a dog's mouth is cleaner than a human's. I know where mine has been, so that can't be good.

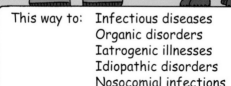

This way to: Infectious diseases
Organic disorders
Iatrogenic illnesses
Idiopathic disorders
Nosocomial infections

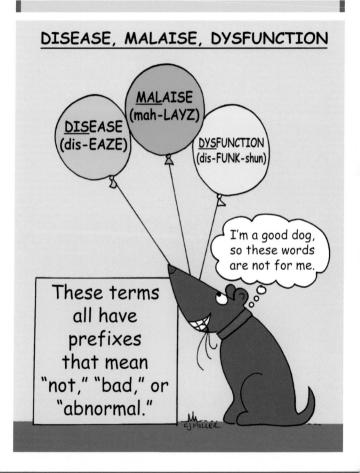

INFECTIOUS DISEASES

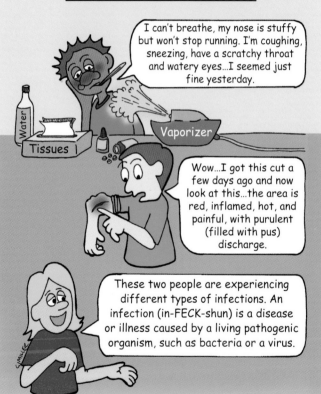

I can't breathe, my nose is stuffy but won't stop running. I'm coughing, sneezing, have a scratchy throat and watery eyes...I seemed just fine yesterday.

Wow...I got this cut a few days ago and now look at this...the area is red, inflamed, hot, and painful, with purulent (filled with pus) discharge.

These two people are experiencing different types of infections. An infection (in-FECK-shun) is a disease or illness caused by a living pathogenic organism, such as bacteria or a virus.

ORGANIC DISORDERS

My garden is organic, but you can also have organic (or-GAN-ick) disorders, which are pathologic conditions with physical changes to explain the symptoms.

That would explain my stomach pain. I have a gastrointestinal ulcer that is destroying my stomach and bowel tissue.

Organically grown

Remember, however, that you don't get organic disorders by eating organically grown foods. They are really good for you.

That's good!

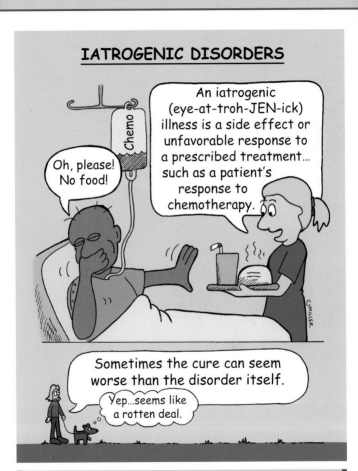

IDIOPATHIC DISORDERS

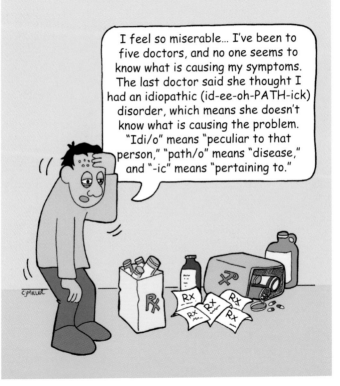

I feel so miserable... I've been to five doctors, and no one seems to know what is causing my symptoms. The last doctor said she thought I had an idiopathic (id-ee-oh-PATH-ick) disorder, which means she doesn't know what is causing the problem. "Idi/o" means "peculiar to that person," "path/o" means "disease," and "-ic" means "pertaining to."

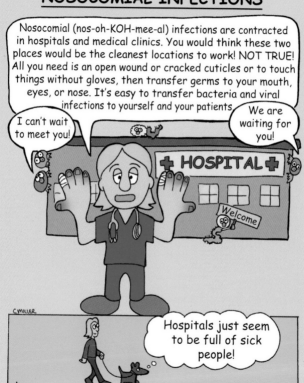

NOSOCOMIAL INFECTIONS

Nosocomial (nos-oh-KOH-mee-al) infections are contracted in hospitals and medical clinics. You would think these two places would be the cleanest locations to work! NOT TRUE! All you need is an open wound or cracked cuticles or to touch things without gloves, then transfer germs to your mouth, eyes, or nose. It's easy to transfer bacteria and viral infections to yourself and your patients.

I can't wait to meet you!

We are waiting for you!

HOSPITAL

Welcome

Hospitals just seem to be full of sick people!

DIAGNOSTIC PROCEDURES

Assessment of the patient means to evaluate the patient's physical and mental condition. Assessment consists of medical professionals using their skills and senses to pick up normal, as well as abnormal, signs and symptoms. The diagnostic procedure starts with the initial assessment with the most advanced technology available to provide the most accurate diagnosis and treatment plan.

Tell me more. I love the way it sounds.

CJMILLER

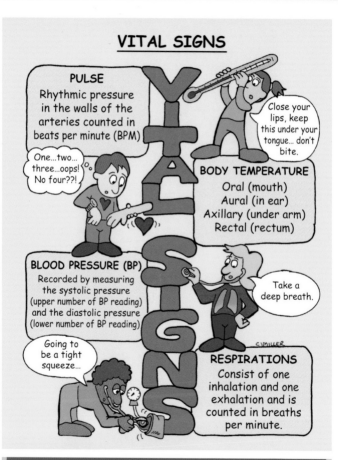

SIGNS, SYMPTOMS, AND SYNDROME

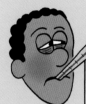

102° F

SIGN

Fever is a sign because it can be measured. It's an objective sign, because it is evaluated with a thermometer.

I have pain and feel tired and weak.

SYMPTOM

Pain, fatigue, and weakness are symptoms (SIMP-tums) and are subjective, which means only the patient can evaluate or measure them.

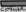

SYNDROME

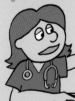

If you have a combination of signs and symptoms that show up together as part of a specific disease process, then you have a syndrome (SIN-drohm).

DIAGNOSIS, DIFFERENTIAL DIAGNOSIS, AND PROGNOSIS

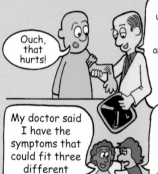

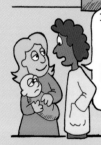

ACUTE, CHRONIC, AND REMISSION

ACUTE

An acute (ah-KYOOT) disorder, such as heartburn, usually has an abrupt onset with intense severity. It ends after a short period.

Heartburn

CHRONIC

A chronic (KRAH-nick) problem is a pain or symptom that has persisted for a long period and is probably not curable.

I have chronic back pain. I've had it since I was thrown from that rodeo bull.

REMISSION

I have liver disease... but I'm in remission. My symptoms have temporarily, partially, or completely disappeared, though I still carry the active disease.

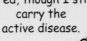

I've been told I'm "ACUTE" DOG.

I'm a survivor

C.MILLER

ASSESSMENT TOOLS

I'm a sphygmomanometer (sfig-moh-mah-NOM-uh-ter). I'm used to measure systolic and diastolic blood pressure levels.

I'm a stethoscope (STETH-oh-skope). I'm used for auscultation (aws-kull-TAY-shun). "Steth/o" means "chest," and "-scope" means an "instrument for examination."

I'm a speculum (SPECK-u-lum). I'm used to enlarge openings of any canal or cavity to facilitate the inspection of its interior, such as with a vaginal speculum.

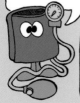

I'm an ophthalmoscope (off-THAL-moh-skope). "Opthalm/o" means "eye," and "-scope" means an "instrument for examination." I'm used to examine the interior of the eye.

I'm an otoscope (oh-TAH-skope). "Ot/o" means "ear," and "-scope" means an "instrument for examination." I'm used to examine the external ear canal and tympanic membrane.

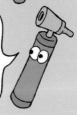

BASIC EXAMINATION POSITIONS

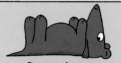

Recumbent
(ree-KUM-bent)

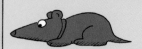

Prone

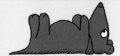

Supine
(SUE-pine or sue-PINE)

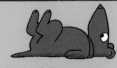

Dorsal Recumbent

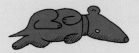

Sims

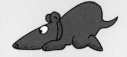

Knee Chest

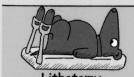

Lithotomy
(lih-THOT-uh-mee)

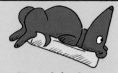

Trendelenburg

LABORATORY TESTS

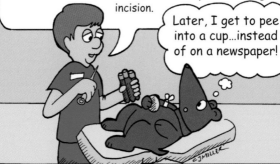

Laboratory tests are conducted on all types of body fluids and cells, such as blood, urine, sputum, stool, and spinal fluid. A phlebotomy (fleh-BOT-uh-me) is done to obtain blood. "Phleb/o" means "vein," and "-tomy" means surgical incision.

Later, I get to pee into a cup...instead of on a newspaper!

Frequently Ordered Blood Tests

Complete blood count (CBC) measures hemoglobin, hematocrit, red blood cells, white blood cells, platelets, and WBC with differential.

Agglutination (ah-GLOO-tih-NAY-shun) **tests** determine blood type compatibility.

Blood urea (yoor-REE-ah) **nitrogen** tests kidney function, also known an BUN.

Prothrombin (proh-THROM-bin) **time** or "protime" diagnoses abnormal bleeding.

URINALYSIS

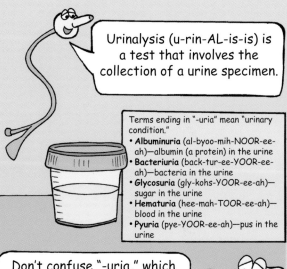

Urinalysis (u-rin-AL-is-is) is a test that involves the collection of a urine specimen.

Terms ending in "-uria" mean "urinary condition."
- **Albuminuria** (al-byoo-mih-NOOR-ee-ah)—albumin (a protein) in the urine
- **Bacteriuria** (back-tur-ee-YOOR-ee-ah)—bacteria in the urine
- **Glycosuria** (gly-kohs-YOOR-ee-ah)—sugar in the urine
- **Hematuria** (hee-mah-TOOR-ee-ah)—blood in the urine
- **Pyuria** (pye-YOOR-ee-ah)—pus in the urine

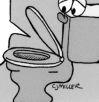

Don't confuse "-uria," which means "urinary condition," with "urea," which is a chemical waste product.

CJMILLER

CENTESIS

Centesis means "surgical puncture to remove fluid."

Tympanocentesis (tim-pah-noh-sen-TEE-sis) is the removal of fluid from behind the eardrum with a special needle with a tube attached to collect the sample of fluid. "Tympan/o" means eardrum.

Thoracentesis (tho-rah-sen-TEE-sis) is the surgical puncture in the pleural space to aspirate fluid from the chest cavity.

Pericardiocentesis (pehr-ih-kar-dee-oh-sen-TEE-sis) is the drawing of fluid from the peri-cardial sac for diagnostic purposes or to relieve pressure. "Peri-" means "around," and "cardi/o" means "heart."

Abdominocentesis (ab-dom-ih-moh-sen-TEE-sis) or paracentesis (par-ah-sen-TEE-sis) is the removal of fluid from the abdomen. "Abdomin/o" means "abdomen," and "para-" means "near" or "beside."

Arthrocentesis (ar-thro-sen-TEE-sis) is the removal of fluid from a joint cavity. "Arthr/o" means "joint."

RADIOLOGY

Different imaging techniques such as x-rays help visualize and examine internal body structures. Radiology uses x-rays to create images of internal structures on specialized film. A radiographic contrast medium is used to make soft organs such as the gastrointestinal tract visible. This medium can be injested or delivered intravenously or via an enema. OK, sir...hold your breath.

I'm supposed to hug this machine, hold still, hold my breath, and relax, all while I watch the radiographer run behind a protective shield. OK...I'm relaxed.

X-ray-o-matic

A doctor who specializes in x-rays is called a radiologist (ray-dee-OL-uh-jist). "Radi/o" means "rays," "log/o" means "knowledge," and "-ist" means "one who is a specialist."

Radical man...

COMPUTERIZED TOMOGRAPHY
OR COMPUTERIZED AXIAL TOMOGRAPHY

(CT or CAT scan)

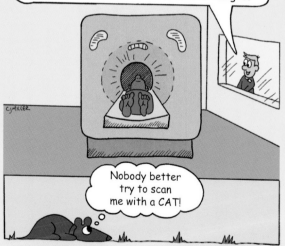

Computerized tomography (toh-MOG-ruh-fee)—
"tom/o" means "cut," "section," or "slice," and
"-graphy" means the "process of recording."
Images are generated by computerized
synthesis of x-ray data (slices or cross-sections)
obtained as the machine rotates around the
client, producing three-dimensional images.

Nobody better
try to scan
me with a CAT!

MAGNETIC RESONANCE IMAGING

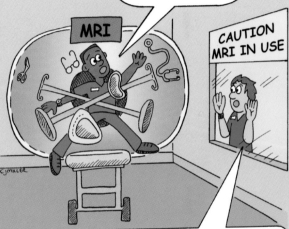

Magnetic resonance imaging (MRI) uses powerful magnetic fields and radiofrequency pulses to produce pictures of the heart, blood vessels, brain, spine, joints, muscles, and internal organs.

FLUOROSCOPY

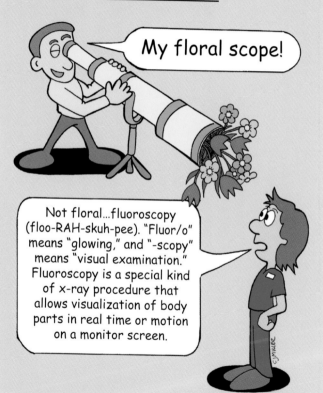

My floral scope!

Not floral...fluoroscopy (floo-RAH-skuh-pee). "Fluor/o" means "glowing," and "-scopy" means "visual examination." Fluoroscopy is a special kind of x-ray procedure that allows visualization of body parts in real time or motion on a monitor screen.

DIAGNOSTIC ULTRASOUND

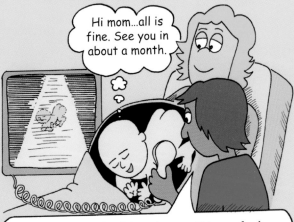

PALLIATIVE MEASURES

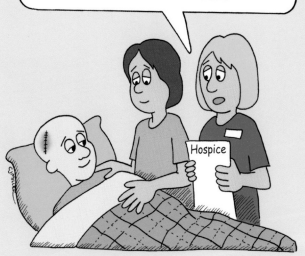

ANTI-, -LYTIC, AND -CIDES

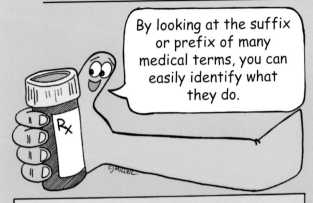

By looking at the suffix or prefix of many medical terms, you can easily identify what they do.

- "Anti-" means "against." An antidepressant is a drug used against depression.

- "-Lytic" mean "to destroy" or "to break down." A hemolytic destroys or breaks down blood (hem/o).

- "-Cide" means "to kill." A germicide is used to kill germs (bacteria).

POTENTIATION AND SYNERGISM

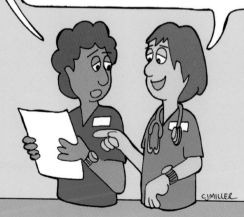

The doctor ordered Demerol and Phenergan for my patient's pain, but Demerol is for pain and Phenergan is for nausea...right?

The potentiation (poh-ten-shee-AY-shun) of Demerol and Phenergan makes them a good combination. The Phenergan enhances Demerol's pain control. It's called "synergism" (SIN-er-jizm) when one drug's effect is increased when combined with another.

DRUG IDIOSYNCRATIC REACTIONS

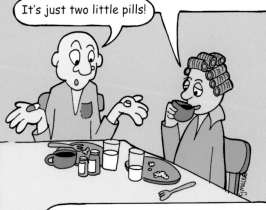

ROUTES OF MEDICATION ADMINISTRATION

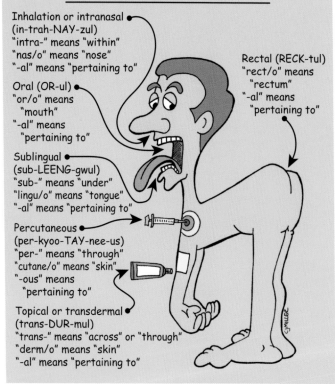

Inhalation or intranasal
(in-trah-NAY-zul)
"intra-" means "within"
"nas/o" means "nose"
"-al" means "pertaining to"

Rectal (RECK-tul)
"rect/o" means
"rectum"
"-al" means
"pertaining to"

Oral (OR-ul)
"or/o" means
"mouth"
"-al" means
"pertaining to"

Sublingual
(sub-LEENG-gwul)
"sub-" means "under"
"lingu/o" means "tongue"
"-al" means "pertaining to"

Percutaneous
(per-kyoo-TAY-nee-us)
"per-" means "through"
"cutane/o" means "skin"
"-ous" means
"pertaining to"

Topical or transdermal
(trans-DUR-mul)
"trans-" means "across" or "through"
"derm/o" means "skin"
"-al" means "pertaining to"

-ECTOMY, -STOMY, AND -TOMY

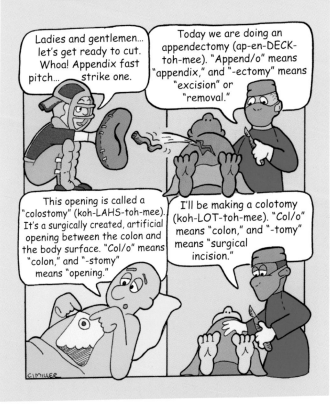

Ladies and gentlemen... let's get ready to cut. Whoa! Appendix fast pitch... strike one.

Today we are doing an appendectomy (ap-en-DECK-toh-mee). "Append/o" means "appendix," and "-ectomy" means "excision" or "removal."

This opening is called a "colostomy" (koh-LAHS-toh-mee). It's a surgically created, artificial opening between the colon and the body surface. "Col/o" means "colon," and "-stomy" means "opening."

I'll be making a colotomy (koh-LOT-toh-mee). "Col/o" means "colon," and "-tomy" means "surgical incision."

Don't Confuse These!

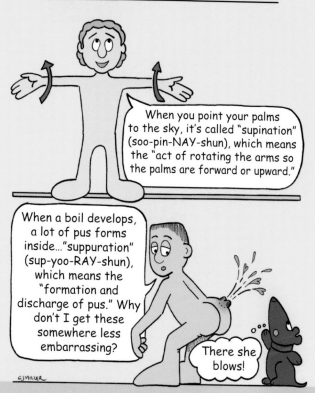

CYT/O AND CYST/O

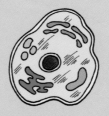

"Cyt/o" refers to a "cell," such as in cytology—the study (-logy) of cells (cyt/o).

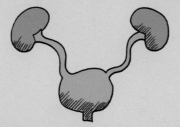

"Cyst/o" refers to a "bladder" or "sac," such as in urinary cystectomy (sis-TECK-tuh-mee)—the excision (-ectomy) of the urinary bladder (cyst/o).

OS AND OSTE/O

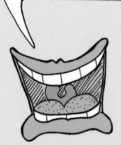

Hi, I'm a mouth. My word part "os" can be easily confused with the combining form "oste/o" for bone... so be careful.

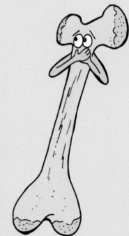

An "os" is any opening, such as "per os," which means "by mouth."

"Osteitis" is an inflammation ("-itis") of the bone ("oste/o").

CJMILLER

SACR/O AND SARC/O

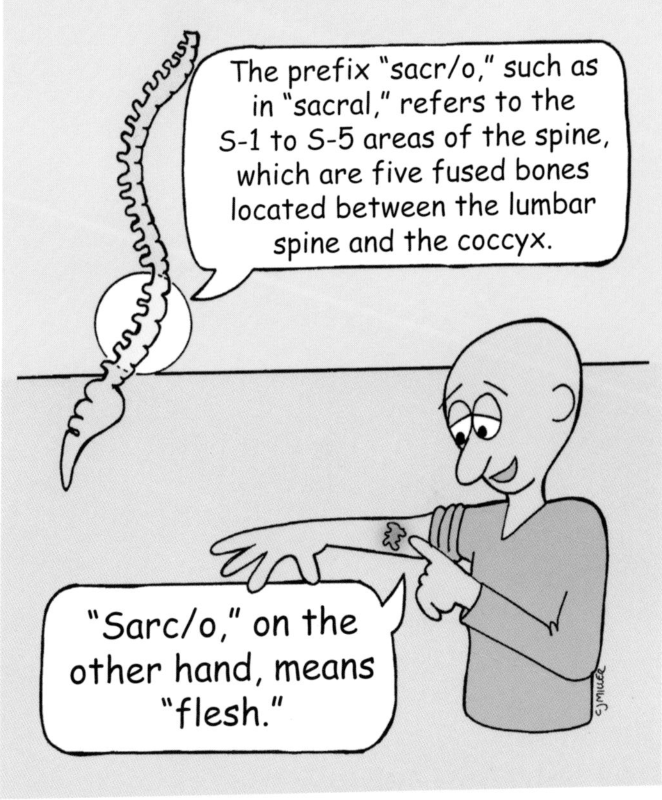

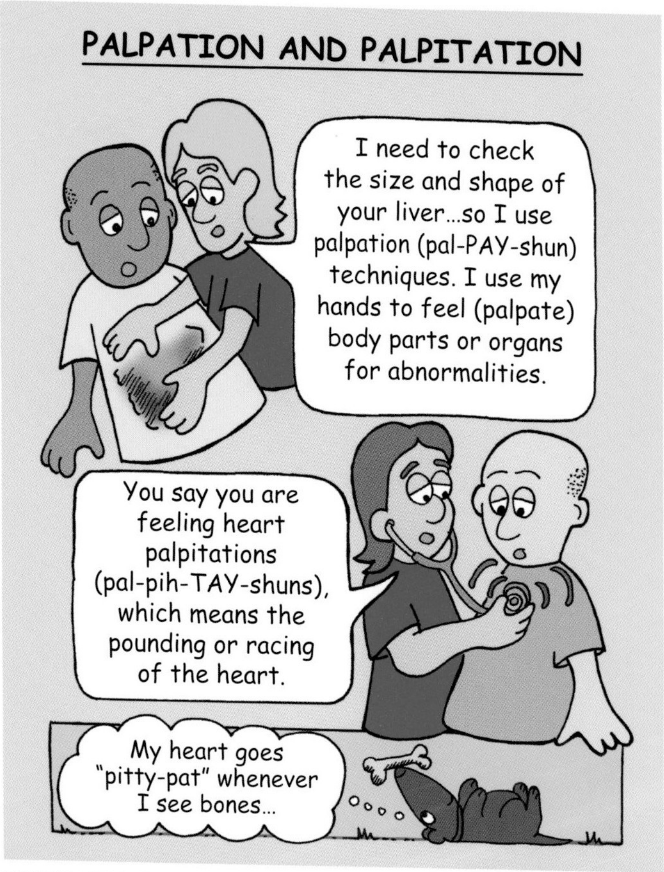
PALPATION AND PALPITATION
I need to check the size and shape of your liver...so I use palpation (pal-PAY-shun) techniques. I use my hands to feel (palpate) body parts or organs for abnormalities.
You say you are feeling heart palpitations (pal-pih-TAY-shuns), which means the pounding or racing of the heart.
My heart goes "pitty-pat" whenever I see bones...

ARTERI/O, ATHER/O, AND ARTHR/O

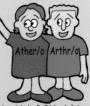

Be careful...these root words may sound alike, <u>but</u> their meanings are specific to situations that may be very different.

Arteriosclerosis (ar-tee-ree-oh-skleh-ROH-sis) is characterized by the thickening and loss of elasticity of the arterial walls. "Arteri/o" means "artery," and "-sclerosis" means "abnormal hardening."

An atheroma (ath-er-OH-ma) is a mass of fat or lipids on an artery wall. "Ather/o" means "plaque" or "fatty substance," and "-oma" means "mass" or "tumor."

Add a suffix as in arthralgia (ar-THRAL-jee-ah), and you get a term that means "joint pain." "Arthr/o" means "joint," and "-algia" means pain.

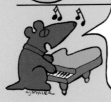

Ooow...I am the artery that lets the red blood flow...the atheroma that makes fatty masses grow. I'm the arthralgia joint pain that makes the whole world cry. I am the dog, I am the dog...or something like that. Take that, Barry!

FISSURE AND FISTULA

FISSURE

A fissure (FISH-ur) can be a fold in the brain tissue or a cracklike lesion (LEE-zhun) of the skin or body.

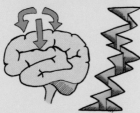

FISTULA

A fistula can be an abnormal passage or channel between two internal organs or from an organ to the surface of the body.

Oh no! It's a fistula (FIST-yoo-lah)! My Crohn's disease has eaten a hole through my colon, and I'm dripping "poo-poo" into my abdominal cavity.

That's bad when even a dog thinks it's gross.

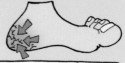

CJMILLER

MYC/O, MYEL/O, AND MY/O

MYC/O

"Mycosis" (my-KOH-sis) means a "disease caused by a fungus." "Myc/o" means "fungus," and "-osis" means "abnormal condition."

MYEL/O

"Myelopathy" (my-eh-LOP-uh-thee) means any "pathologic change in the bone marrow or spinal cord." "Myel/o" means "spinal cord" or "bone marrow," and "-pathy" means "disease."

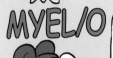

Buddy...drop the bone.

MY/O

"My/o" means "muscle," and "-pathy" means "disease." Sooo, "myopathy" (my-OP-uh-thee) would mean a "muscle disease..." Cool huh!

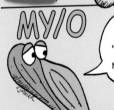

Don't Confuse These!

ILEUM AND ILIUM

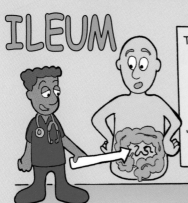

ILEUM

The ileum (ILL-ee-um) is the area of the small intestine that attaches to the colon. Remember, when you see ileum with an "e," think "enter/o," which means "small intestine."

ILIUM

The ilium (ILL-ee-um) is a part of the hip bone, and the word is spelled with an "i." Remember, there is an "i" in hip...just like ilium.

CJMILLER

PYEL/O, PY/O, AND PYR/O

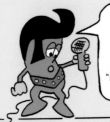

"Pyel/o" means "renal pelvis," a part of the kidneys. So, if I had an inflammation in my renal pelvic area, it would be called "pyelonephritis" (pye-uh-loh-neh-FRY-tis) "Pyel/o" means "renal pelvis," "nephr/o" means "kidney," and "-itis" means inflammation. Thank you, thank you very much.

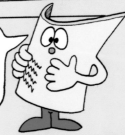

The doctor told me that my wound is inflamed, draining, and infected. He called the wound "pyoderma" (pye-oh-DER-mah). "Py/o" means "pus," and "-derma" means "skin."

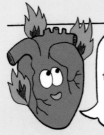

"Pyr/o" means "fever" or "fire." So...pyrosis (pye-ROH-sis) is made from the words "pyr/o" meaning "fever" or "fire" and "-sis" meaning "abnormal condition." This is also known as "heartburn."

Don't Confuse These!

PERONE/O, PERINE/O, AND PERITONE/O

"Perone/o" refers to the fibula, the outer, smaller bone in the lower leg. The word "peroneal" means "concerning the fibula" (FIB-yuh-luh).

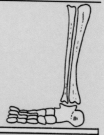

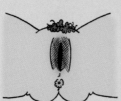

"Perine/o" refers to the space between the external genitalia and the anus. This space is called the "perineum" (pair-ih-NEE-um).

"Peritone/o" refers to the lining of the abdominal cavity. This lining is called the "peritoneum" (pair-uh-tuh-NEE-um).

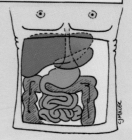

PHALL/O AND PHALANG/O

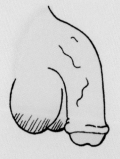

"Phall/o" means "penis" (PEE-nuss), such as in the word "phallorrhagia" (fal-oh-RAH-jah), which means "bleeding" (-rrhagia) "from the penis" (phall/o).

CJMILLER

"Phalang/o" means the "bones of the fingers or toes," such as in the word "phalangitis" (fay-lan-JI-tis), which means "inflammation" (-itis) "of the bones of the fingers or toes" (phalang/o).

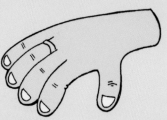

Don't Confuse These!

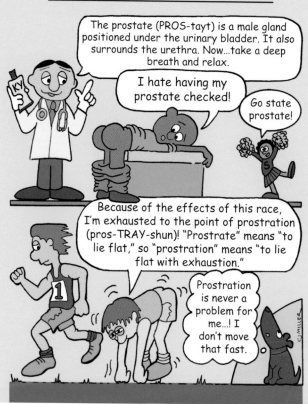

VESIC/O AND VESICUL/O

Vesic/o refers to the urinary bladder, such as in the word "vesicotomy" (vess-ih-KAH-tuh-mee), which means "making an incision" (-tomy) "into the bladder" (vesic/o).

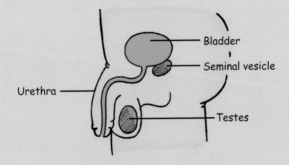

Vesicul/o refers to the seminal vesicle, such as in the word "vesiculitis" (veh-sick-yoo-LYE-tis), which means "inflammation" (-itis) "of the seminal vesicle" (vesicul/o).

CJ MILLER

Don't Confuse These!

VIRAL AND VIRILE

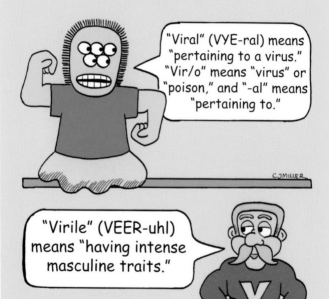

"Viral" (VYE-ral) means "pertaining to a virus." "Vir/o" means "virus" or "poison," and "-al" means "pertaining to."

"Virile" (VEER-uhl) means "having intense masculine traits."

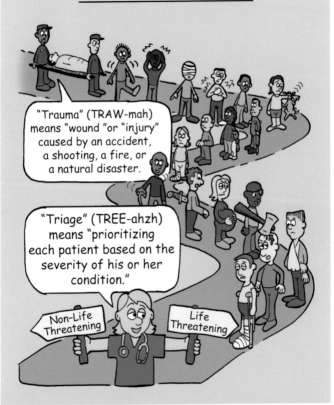

Don't Confuse These!

A